HIV/AIDS and the Eye

A Global Perspective

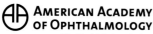

HIV/AIDS and the Eye

A Global Perspective

Emmett T. Cunningham, Jr, MD, PhD, MPH

The Francis I. Proctor Foundation
University of California, San Francisco

Rubens Belfort, Jr, MD, PhD, MBA

Department of Ophthalmology
Federal University of São Paulo, Brazil

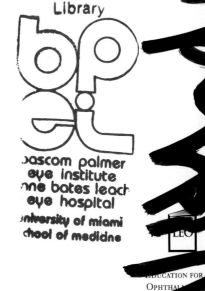

Norto
Library

bp
ei

bascom palmer
eye institute
anne bates leach
eye hospital

university of miami
school of medicine

LEO

EDUCATION FOR T
OPHTHAL   ST

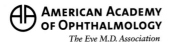

**AMERICAN ACADEMY
OF OPHTHALMOLOGY**

The Eye M.D. Association

LIFELONG
EDUCATION FOR THE
OPHTHALMOLOGIST®

Ophthalmology Monograph 15, *HIV/AIDS and the Eye: A Global Perspective*, is one component of the Lifelong Education for the Ophthalmologist (LEO) framework, which assists members in planning their continuing medical education. LEO includes an array of clinical education products and programs that members may select to form individualized, self-directed learning plans for updating their clinical knowledge. Active members or fellows who use LEO components may accumulate sufficient CME credits to earn the LEO Award. Contact the Academy's Clinical Education Division for further information on LEO.

This work is published by the Clinical Education Division
of the Foundation of the American Academy of Ophthalmology,
a 501(c)(3) sub-fund.

Library of Congress Cataloging-in-Publication Data

Cunningham, Emmett T.
    HIV/AIDS and the eye : a global perspective / Emmett T. Cunningham, Jr., Rubens
Belfort, Jr.
        p. ; cm. — (Ophthalmology monographs ; 15) (Lifelong education for the ophthalmologist)
    includes bibliographical references and index.
    ISBN 1-56055-264-6
        1. Eye—Infections. 2. AIDS (Disease)—Complications. 3. Ocular manifestations of
general diseases. I. Belfort, R. (Rubens) II. American Academy of Ophthalmology. III.
Title. IV. Series. V. Series: Lifelong education for the ophthalmologist
        [DNLM: 1. HIV Infections—prevention & control. 2. Acquired Immunodeficiency
Syndrome—prevention & control. 3. Disease Transmission, Patient-to-Professional. 4.
Eye Manifestations. 5. Opportunistic Infections. WC 503.6 C973h 2002]
    RE96.C865 2002
    617.7'1—dc21
                                                                    2001053612

07 06 05 04 03   5 4 3 2 1

Printed in Singapore

**To the millions of patients who have suffered
from the ravages of HIV/AIDS**

Contents

Preface

HIV/AIDS affects millions of people worldwide, and the vast majority of individuals infected with HIV will, at some point, develop ocular complications related to their disease. We hope, therefore, that a concise summary of the key issues related to HIV/AIDS and the eye will be useful to people who care for HIV-infected patients, particularly those whose job it is to diagnosis and manage the ocular complications associated with HIV disease.

The care of patients with HIV/AIDS is both complex and multifaceted. In fact, HIV-positive patients typically have teams of doctors, including both generalists and specialists. The material presented in this monograph is thus intended to be accessible to eye care providers and general practitioners alike. In addition, we strove throughout the monograph to provide practical, clinically relevant information. We also tried to maintain a global perspective, both because the vast majority of HIV-infected individuals live in nations with limited economic and health care resources and because globalization is quickly blurring the distinctions between the developed nations and the developing countries of the world.

The educational objectives of this monograph are to

- Review the global epidemiology of HIV/AIDS

- Explain the molecular biology of HIV

- Discuss the pathogenesis of AIDS

- Provide an overview of HIV transmission and prophylaxis

- Summarize the key issues related to the diagnosis and management of the ocular complications of HIV/AIDS

Emmett T. Cunningham, Jr, MD, PhD, MPH
Rubens Belfort, Jr, MD, PhD, MBA

CHAPTER 1

Epidemiology

The human immunodeficiency virus (HIV) almost certainly spread from nonhuman primates to humans somewhere in central Africa. Human infections appear to have been sporadic and limited to Africa until the 1970s, when international travel and the practice of unprotected sexual intercourse and intravenous drug use fueled rapid expansion of regional epidemics in Africa, the Americas, and Western Europe. The first cases of what is now recognized as the acquired immunodeficiency syndrome (AIDS) were reported from Los Angeles in 1981. HIV itself was isolated shortly thereafter by independent investigators in France and the United States in 1983 and 1984, respectively.

Over the past 20 years, HIV outbreaks have occurred in literally thousands of communities throughout the world, producing a pandemic of enormous proportions. Recent estimates from the Joint United Nations Programme on HIV/AIDS (UNAIDS) and the World Health Organization (WHO) suggest that since the early 1980s, more than 50 million people have been infected with HIV around the world and that, globally, HIV has caused nearly 22 million deaths and left more than 13 million orphans. These same estimates suggest that 10 to 15 men, women, and children are infected with HIV each minute, resulting in a staggering 15,000 to 20,000 new infections each day. To compound matters, the vast majority of people infected with HIV live in developing nations, those countries least able to afford the enormous social and financial costs of caring for those who are infected. It is estimated that less than 10% of HIV-positive people in the developing world are aware that they are infected.

1-1

RISK FACTORS AND TRANSMISSION

HIV resides and replicates primarily in CD4$^+$ T lymphocytes, a T-cell subset critical for antigen-dependent immune activation (Figure 1-1). The risk of transmission is therefore greatest with exposure to contaminated blood or blood products, but can, theoretically, occur following exposure to any contaminated body fluid, including semen, breast milk, saliva, and tears. High-risk activities include unprotected sexual intercourse, particularly men having sex with men, injection drug use (IDU), and receipt of blood and blood products, most often by transfusion. Children born to HIV-infected women are also at greatly increased risk of infection.

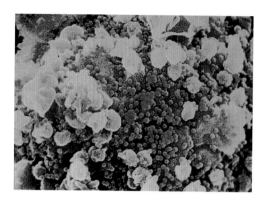

Figure 1-1 *CD4+ T lymphocyte actively infected with HIV. Numerous viral particles, here pseudocolored green, are seen budding from cell surface.*
Reproduced with permission from Greene WC: AIDS and the immune system. Sci Am *1993;269:98–105.*

1-1-1 Sexual Transmission

In North America and Europe, the majority of HIV-positive patients are either homosexual or bisexual men. Risk factors in this group include receptive anal intercourse, a high number of sexual partners, rectal trauma, or a history of an ulcerating anogenital infection, as might occur with gonorrhea, syphilis, or herpes simplex virus. Transmission may also occur following orogenital sex, but the risk appears to be much lower.

Worldwide, the majority of HIV transmission occurs heterosexually. This route of transmission is also increasing in North America and Europe, particularly among women and minorities. Risk factors include multiple sex partners, unprotected intercourse with commercial sex workers, sex with IDU, or a history of sexually transmitted disease. Latex condoms are an inexpensive and effective barrier against HIV transmission when used consistently and correctly.

1-1-2 Injection Drug Use Transmission

Injection drug use is a major risk factor for the transmission of HIV, particularly among minorities and women. In some cities along the East Coast of the United States, in Puerto Rico, and in parts of Southeast Asia, South America, Eastern Europe, and the former Soviet Union, one third to one half of all HIV-positive patients are infected by contaminated needles or other paraphernalia used during IDU. In most regions, however, IDU accounts for less than 10% of all HIV-positive cases. Needle-sharing appears to be the primary mode of transmission, although this route may be amplified by un-protected sex and sexually transmitted dis-eases in this population. Children born to women who practice IDU are also at in-creased risk of HIV infection.

1-1-3 Blood and Blood Products Transmission

Receipt of HIV-contaminated blood or blood products, and of organs transplanted from HIV-positive patients, is associated with a rate of seroconversion that ap-proaches 100%. Fortunately, however, in-fection by these routes is now extremely rare in most developed nations. This is due in large part to self-deferral of potential donors who are known to be either infected or at high risk of infection, improved donor interviewing regarding high-risk behaviors, maintenance of regularly updated donor de-ferral lists, and routine use of sensitive and specific HIV antibody screening tests. In countries where such practices are not em-ployed, however, the risk of infection asso-ciated with receiving blood, blood products, or whole organs can be high.

1-1-4 Prenatal and Postnatal Transmission

Mother-to-child transmission of HIV ac-counts for over 90% of the more than 1.4 million children currently living with HIV/ AIDS worldwide. Such vertical transmis-sion may occur prepartum, intrapartum, or postpartum by way of breast-feeding. Intra-partum transmission probably accounts for the greatest number of infections, although up to 15% of HIV-infected children are believed to have seroconverted following breast-feeding.

Rates of mother-to-child transmission vary from approximately 15% in Europe, to 20% to 30% in the United States, to as high as 50% in some African countries. The rea-sons for such wide variations are not en-tirely known, but are most probably related to regional differences in the use of anti-retroviral agents and/or the prevalence or duration of breast-feeding. The risk of transmission appears to be higher with advanced HIV disease and lower $CD4^+$ T-lymphocyte counts in the mother. The transmission rate may be lowered dramati-cally by treating both the mother and the child with antiretroviral agents before, dur-ing, and after delivery.

1-1-5 Transmission to and from Health Care Workers

Fortunately, transmission from HIV-posi-tive patients to health care workers or from HIV-positive health care workers to pa-tients is extremely uncommon. When last reported in June of 1997, the Centers for Disease Control and Prevention (CDC) had received reports from various centers in the United States of 52 HIV seroconversions in health care workers that were temporally correlated with known occupational HIV exposures, as well as an additional 114 re-ports that were considered possible occupational HIV transmissions. The vast majority of these seroconversions occurred following percutaneous exposure to either blood or visibly bloody fluid, and the CDC has estimated the risk of HIV infection following such exposure to be about 0.3%, compared to the 0.1% probability of seroconverting following male-to-female sexual intercourse. Very few cases, in contrast, have been reported following mucocutaneous exposure. Moreover, according to the CDC, more than 80% of these health care workers experienced systemic symptoms consistent with primary HIV infection within 1 month of exposure. Seroconversion occurred in more than 50% of exposed patients within 2 months (median 46 days, mean 65 days) and in more than 95% within 6 months. Seroconversions occurring after 6 months were uncommon.

Only two reports of HIV transmission from infected health care workers to patients have appeared in the literature. One report involved a surgeon who infected a cluster of 6 patients. The second report involved transmission from a dentist to his patients. The routes of transmission in these cases remain unknown and, in general, provider-to-patient transmission is believed to be extremely rare.

To date, no seroconversions in health care workers have been associated with exposure to saliva, tears, sweat, or nonbloody urine or feces from HIV-infected patients. This, of course, should not minimize the importance of using appropriately protective eye shields or latex gloves when handling potentially infected body fluids or of routine hand-washing as part of standard infection control and prevention (discussed in Chapter 3, "Prevention of HIV Transmission"). In fact, a case of HIV transmission has been reported following ocular contamination by infected serum droplets.

Postexposure antiretroviral therapy is generally advised for occupational exposures in which there is a recognized transmission risk. Specific treatment guidelines change often, however, as new antiretroviral agents become available. Current recommendations may be obtained either from the HIV/AIDS National Clinicians Consultation Center, located at San Francisco General Hospital (1-888-448-4911), or from institutional infection control centers.

1-2

PROGRESSION OF INFECTION

The natural history of untreated HIV infection may be somewhat artificially divided into three phases (Figure 1-2): (1) a first phase of primary infection; (2) a second phase of clinical latency; and (3) a third phase characterized by the development of opportunistic infections and neoplasms, also referred to as *AIDS*.

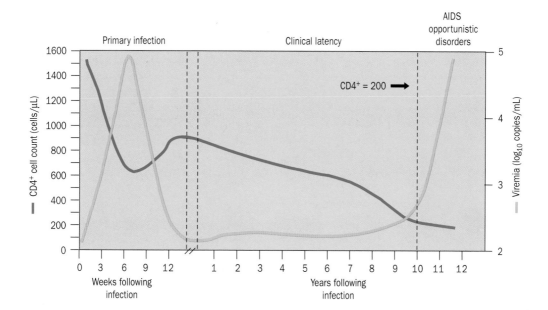

1. Primary HIV infection produces a burst of viral replication and widespread lysis of infected T lymphocytes and monocytes. These events produce an intense viremia, a decrease in circulating CD4⁺ T lymphocytes, and, in most patients, a moderately severe flu-like illness 2 to 4 weeks after inoculation. Common symptoms include fever, lymphadenopathy, rash, pharyngitis, headache, nausea, and diarrhea. An HIV-specific cytotoxic T-lymphocyte response and seroconversion result within 4 to 8 weeks. These result in a decrease in circulating HIV and allow rapid, albeit partial, repletion of peripheral CD4⁺ T lymphocytes.

2. Clinical latency follows primary infection and lasts for at least 10 years in 25% to 50% of untreated patients. During this time, viral replication continues in both reticulo-

Figure 1-2 *Natural history of untreated HIV infection. Clinical phases include primary infection, clinical latency, and AIDS. CDC defines AIDS as occurrence of opportunistic infection or neoplasm or CD4⁺ T-lymphocyte count of <200 cells/μL.*

Modified with permission of American College of Physicians–American Society of Internal Medicine from Fauci AS, Pantaleo G, Stanley S, et al: Immunopathogenic mechanisms of HIV infection. Ann Intern Med 1996;124:654–663.

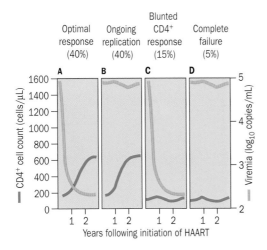

Figure 1-3 *Possible CD4⁺ T-lymphocyte and viral-load responses to HAART in patients with AIDS. (A) Approximately 40% of patients experience optimal response, including increased CD4⁺ T-lymphocyte counts and marked viral suppression. (B) Another 40% of patients experience increased CD4⁺ cell counts despite ongoing viral replication. (C) Approximately 15% of patients experience blunted CD4⁺ cell-count response despite viral control. (D) Up to 5% of patients experience complete treatment failure. Predictors of treatment failure are incompletely understood, but appear to include poor adherence to HAART, prior exposure to antiretroviral medications as single or dual therapy, sequential addition of drugs to failing regimen, and adverse interactions between drugs used.*

Modified with permission from Perrin L, Telenti A: HIV treatment failure: testing for HIV resistance in clinical practice. Science 1998;280:1871–1873. Copyright 1998 American Association for the Advancement of Science.

endothelial tissue and in peripheral lymphocytes, but may be low or difficult to measure in plasma. CD4⁺ T-lymphocyte counts continue to decline, and many patients develop symptoms suggestive of impaired T-cell immunity, including generalized lymphadenopathy, recurrent fevers, night sweats, malaise, mucosal candidiasis, and herpes zoster dermatitis (shingles). The best predictor for rapid progression appears to be a high viral load.

3. The end result of continued HIV replication is AIDS. Lymph node architecture is disrupted, CD4⁺ T lymphocytes approach near-total depletion, and circulating virus levels climb as the patient's ability to combat the infection fails. With this comes a greatly increased susceptibility to a number of infections and neoplasms, many of which can produce vision loss, either by directly affecting the eye or its surrounding structures or by affecting the brain.

The advent in 1996 of highly active antiretroviral therapy (HAART), a combination of three or more antiretroviral agents, including a protease inhibitor, has altered the natural history of HIV infection in two very important ways:

1. Patients are living longer with higher CD4⁺ T-lymphocyte counts and lower, or even undetectable, viral loads.

2. Some patients with pre-existing CD4⁺ T-lymphocyte depletion are experiencing immune reconstitution, including reduced viral loads, significant and sustained elevations in circulating CD4⁺ cell counts (Figure 1-3), and a regained immunologic ability to control opportunistic infections and neoplasms.

Throughout both immune depletion and reconstitution, total CD4$^+$ T-lymphocyte count appears to be a reliable predictor of the risk of AIDS-associated ocular complications for most patients. Whereas some opportunistic disorders, such as Kaposi sarcoma, lymphoma, and herpes zoster ophthalmicus, can occur in the setting of modest CD4$^+$ count depression, others, such as HIV retinopathy, cytomegalovirus (CMV) retinitis, varicella zoster virus (VZV) retinitis, and microsporidial keratitis, require profound levels of T-cell depletion (Table 1-1; see Figure 1-2). High viral loads are a predictor of rapid disease progression independent of CD4$^+$ cell counts.

TABLE 1-1

Ophthalmic Manifestations of HIV Infection by CD4$^+$ T-Lymphocyte Count

CD4$^+$ T-Lymphocyte Count, cells/μL	Complication
<500	Herpes zoster ophthalmicus
	Kaposi sarcoma
	Lymphoma
<200	Coccidioidomycosis
	Cryptococcosis
	Histoplasmosis
	Pneumocystosis
	Toxoplasmosis
	Tuberculosis
<100	Cytomegalovirus retinitis
	Microsporidiosis
	Mycobacterium avium complex infection
	Progressive multifocal leukoencephalopathy
	Retinal/conjunctival microvasculopathy
	Varicella zoster virus retinitis

Sources: *Modified with permission from Bartlett JG:* The Johns Hopkins Hospital 1998–1999 Guide to Medical Care of Patients With HIV Infection. *8th ed. Baltimore, MD: Williams & Wilkins; 1999.*

Cunningham ET Jr, Margolis TP: Ocular manifestations of HIV infection. N Engl J Med 1998;339:236–244. Copyright © 1998 Massachusetts Medical Society. All rights reserved.

TESTING AND COUNSELING

HIV testing is essential for long-term prevention and treatment of HIV-related disease. In the United States, HIV testing is mandatory for military recruits, prisoners, immigrants, and blood donors. For most patients, however, testing is voluntary and should be done only after obtaining an appropriately informed consent. There are many relative indications for testing, including documented high-risk sexual behavior or IDU, receipt of blood, blood products, or an organ transplant, especially between 1978 and 1985, or the occurrence of what would be considered an opportunistic infection or neoplasm.

The physician requesting the test should take care to justify the test and to explain to the patient in advance the implications of positive, negative, and indeterminate results. This discussion should include an absolute assurance of privacy and confidentiality. HIV test results are best reported directly to the patient at a return office visit, because denial, anger, remorse, depression, and even suicide can all be triggered by a positive HIV test result. The physician should be prepared, at this visit, to present the patient with HIV-related educational information, including information for future risk reduction and, in the case of a positive result, counseling, support, and treatment options.

A number of techniques are now available for detecting HIV in patients at risk of infection, including virus culture, antibody detection, antigen detection, and viral DNA and RNA amplification. Serum antibody tests, including the standard enzyme-linked immunosorbent assay (ELISA) and the Western blot, are employed most commonly in routine clinical practice. In general, the ELISA is used as a first screening test, whereas the Western blot is confirmatory. While both tests are extremely sensitive and specific, false-negatives can occur, particularly during the first few months

after infection or following recent blood transfusion or bone marrow transplantation. Similarly, false-positive results can also occur, especially when testing is applied to patients or populations not thought to be at increased risk. This is because the probability of a positive test result occurring in a truly infected individual is critically dependent on the prevalence of HIV infection in the population being tested.

Assume, for example, that only 1 in 1000 people in a given population is HIV-positive and that the sensitivity and specificity of a given HIV antibody test are each 99.9%. These might seem like exceptionally good sensitivity and specificity parameters, and indeed they are, because 99.9% sensitivity will almost always permit the identification of the 1 truly positive patient among the 1000 living in the hypothetical population. The downside, however, is that the 99.9% specificity also produces roughly 1 false-positive patient in this group of 1000. Hence, randomly testing 1000 people yields two positive results: one true and the other false. The chance that either result is truly positive is, therefore, only 50%, or exactly equivalent to flipping a coin. If, however, the population tested has a 5% true HIV seropositivity rate, then testing 1000 consecutive people would, on average, produce 50 positive results, of which roughly 49 would be true positives. This would make the chance that any particular positive result was true approximately 98%. The message, therefore, is that testing should be pursued only in patients thought to be at increased risk of HIV infection.

Once a patient is found to be HIV-positive, other tests, especially viral load and CD4$^+$ T-lymphocyte count, become increasingly important for initiating and monitoring response to treatment, for tracking disease progression, and for assessing a patient's risk for HIV-associated disorders.

1-4

AIDS DEFINITIONS

AIDS is characterized by the occurrence of opportunistic infections and neoplasms. The frequency of opportunistic disorders increases in HIV-positive patients as their CD4$^+$ T-lymphocyte counts decline. For this reason, the CDC expanded its definition of AIDS in 1993 to include either the presence of an AIDS-defining illness (Table 1-2) or a CD4$^+$ count of less than 200 cells/µL.

The WHO definition of AIDS, which is also used by the European Centre for the Epidemiological Monitoring of AIDS (CESES), differs from the CDC definition of AIDS primarily in that it does not include CD4$^+$ T-lymphocyte count. This results in somewhat lower prevalence estimates of AIDS in Europe than might otherwise be expected if the CDC definition were used. For children under 13 years of age, the WHO and European case definition of AIDS is essentially the same as that used in the United States (discussed in Chapter 8, "Manifestations in Children").

TABLE 1-2

Conditions Included in Centers for Disease Control and Prevention 1993 Revised AIDS Surveillance Case Definition

Candidiasis of bronchi, trachea, or lungs

Candidiasis of esophagus

Coccidioidomycosis, disseminated or extrapulmonary

Cryptococcosis, extrapulmonary

Cryptosporidiosis, chronic intestinal (>1 month)

Cytomegalovirus disease (other than liver, spleen, or lymph nodes)

Cytomegalovirus retinitis

Encephalopathy, HIV-related

Herpes simplex virus, chronic ulcer(s) (>1 month), or bronchitis, pneumonitis, or esophagitis

Histoplasmosis, disseminated or extrapulmonary

Isosporiasis, chronic intestinal (>1 month)

Kaposi sarcoma

Lymphoma, Burkitt (or equivalent term)

Lymphoma, immunoblastic (or equivalent term)

Lymphoma, primary central nervous system

Mycobacterium avium complex or *M kansasii*, disseminated or extrapulmonary

Mycobacterium tuberculosis, any site

Pneumocystis carinii pneumonia

Pneumonia, recurrent

Progressive multifocal leukoencephalopathy

Salmonella sp septicemia, recurrent

Toxoplasmosis of central nervous system

Wasting syndrome caused by HIV infection

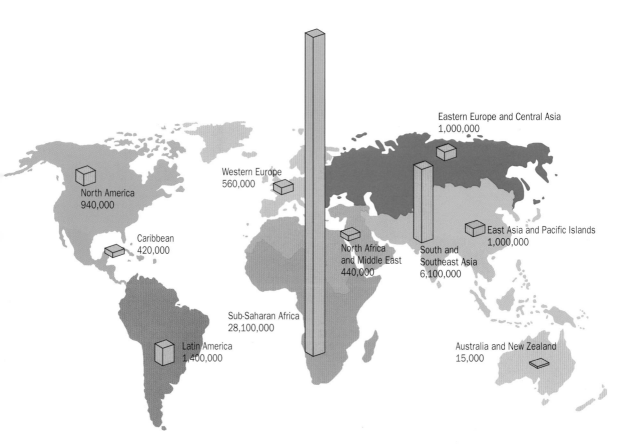

Figure 1-4 *People living with HIV/AIDS in various regions as of December 2001.*

Modified with permission from Mann JM, Tarantola DJ: HIV 1998: the global picture. Sci Am *1998;279:82–83. Data taken from Joint United Nations Programme on HIV/AIDS:* AIDS Epidemic Update. *Geneva: UNAIDS; December 2001.*

1-5

GLOBAL TRENDS

The Joint United Nations Programme on HIV/AIDS (UNAIDS) provides an annual update on the global epidemiology of HIV infection and AIDS (www.unaids.org). The prevalence, incidence, and demographics of HIV/AIDS change quickly and vary dramatically from region to region. Asia, Eastern Europe, and southern Africa are currently experiencing the most rapid rise in infection rates. Statistics as of December 2000 and 2001 for some of the most severely affected regions are summarized below (Figures 1-4 and 1-5; Tables 1-3 and 1-4).

1-5-1 North America and Western Europe

HAART has reduced dramatically the number of new AIDS cases and of AIDS-related deaths in North America, Western Europe,

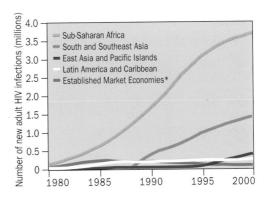

Figure 1-5 *People infected with HIV in various regions over time. *North America, Western Europe, Japan, Australia, and New Zealand.*

Modified with permission from Mann JM, Tarantola DJ: HIV 1998: the global picture. Sci Am 1998;279:82–83. Data taken from Joint United Nations Programme on HIV/AIDS: AIDS Epidemic Update. Geneva: UNAIDS; December 2000.

TABLE 1-3

Global Summary of HIV/AIDS Epidemic, December 2001 (millions)

	Total	Adults	Women	Children <15 Years
People newly infected during 2001	5.0	4.3	1.8	0.8
People living with HIV/AIDS	40.0	37.2	17.6	2.7
AIDS deaths during 2001	3.0	2.4	1.1	0.6
Total AIDS deaths since 1980	21.8	17.5	9.0	4.3

Source: *Joint United Nations Programme on HIV/AIDS: AIDS Epidemic Update. Geneva: UNAIDS; December 2001.*

TABLE 1-4

Regional HIV/AIDS Statistics and Features, December 2001

Region	Epidemic Started	Adults and Children Living With HIV/AIDS	Adults and Children Newly Infected With HIV	Adult Prevalence Rate*	Percentage of HIV-Positive Adult Women	Main Modes[†] of Spread Among Adults
North America	Late 1970s Early 1980s	940,000	45,000	0.6%	20%	MSM IDU MSW
Western Europe	Late 1970s Early 1980s	560,000	30,000	0.3%	25%	MSM IDU
Eastern Europe and Central Asia	Early 1990s	1 million	250,000	0.5%	20%	IDU
Latin America	Late 1970s Early 1980s	1.4 million	130,000	0.5%	30%	MSM IDU MSW
Australia and New Zealand	Late 1970s Early 1980s	15,000	500	0.1%	10%	MSM
East Asia and Pacific Islands	Late 1980s	1 million	270,000	0.1%	20%	IDU MSW MSM
Caribbean	Late 1970s Early 1980s	420,000	60,000	2.2%	50%	MSW MSM
South and Southeast Asia	Late 1980s	6.1 million	800,000	0.6%	35%	MSW IDU
North Africa and Middle East	Late 1980s	440,000	80,000	0.2%	40%	MSW IDU
Sub-Saharan Africa	Late 1970s Early 1980s	28.1 million	3.4 million	8.4%	55%	MSW
Total		**40 million**	**5 million**	**1.2%**	**48%**	

*Proportion of adults (defined as 15 to 49 years of age) living with HIV/AIDS in 2001, using 2001 population numbers.
[†]IDU = injection drug use. MSM = men having sex with men. MSW = men having sex with women.
Source: *Joint United Nations Programme on HIV/AIDS:* AIDS Epidemic Update. *Geneva: UNAIDS; December 2001.*

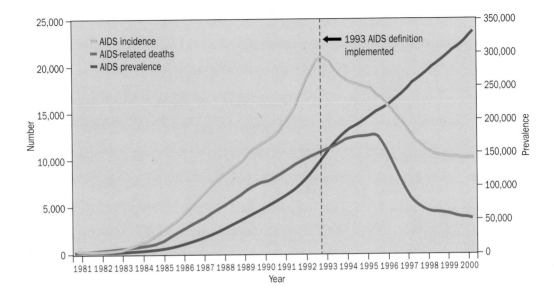

Figure 1-6 *Estimated AIDS incidence, AIDS-related deaths, and prevalence of AIDS by year of diagnosis/ death in United States, 1981–2000. Although incidence of AIDS and number of AIDS-related deaths have both been decreasing in recent years due in large part to introduction of HAART, combination of increased survival and ongoing infection with HIV has resulted in steady increase in prevalence of AIDS.*

Modified from Centers for Disease Control and Prevention: The global HIV and AIDS epidemic, 2001. MMWR *2001; 50:434–439.*

and other parts of the world. Still, new infections continue to occur, particularly among injection drug users and heterosexuals. This combination of increased survival and ongoing infection has resulted in many more people living with HIV/AIDS (Figure 1-6), a number that now approaches 1 million in North America and exceeds 500,000 in Western Europe.

While the number of AIDS cases among homosexuals, bisexuals, and injection drug users in the United States has been decreasing in recent years, the epidemic appears to be growing among heterosexuals (Figure 1-7), particularly among heterosexual minorities and women. AIDS is now the leading killer in African-American men and women aged 25 to 44 and the third leading cause of death in women overall in this age group. In fact, nearly 80% of HIV-infected women in the United States are either African-American or Hispanic. Heterosex-

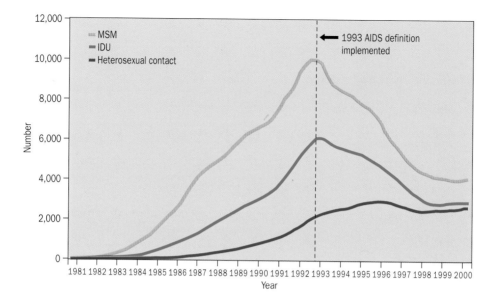

Figure 1-7 *Number of AIDS cases among men who have sex with men (MSM), injection drug users (IDU), and persons exposed through heterosexual contact by year of diagnosis in United States, 1981–2000. Although number of AIDS cases among MSM and IDU has been decreasing in recent years, epidemic appears to be growing among heterosexuals, particularly among minorities and women.*

Modified from Centers for Disease Control and Prevention: The global HIV and AIDS epidemic, 2001. MMWR 2001; 50:434–439.

ual transmission has now surpassed homosexual transmission as the predominant mode of infection in several European countries as well, including France, Norway, and Sweden.

1-5-2 Eastern Europe and Central Asia

An epidemic of HIV infection has exploded in Eastern Europe and Central Asia since 1995, with HIV seropositivity rates climbing between 6- and 7-fold in many countries. Ukraine has been most affected, although Russia, Belarus, and Moldova have recorded staggering increases in HIV positivity as well. Although the epidemic appears to have entered Eastern Europe and Central Asia primarily through IDU, HIV infection is increasing rapidly among homosexual men and heterosexual men and women in most countries in these regions.

1-5-3 Latin America and the Caribbean

The epidemiology of HIV infection in many parts of Latin America, including Mexico, parallels that in industrialized countries. Most transmission occurs in men who have unprotected sex with other men, although IDU accounts for a significant number of HIV-positive patients, particularly in Brazil, Argentina, and Chile. Heterosexual transmission is on the rise in many Latin American countries. This is particularly true in Brazil, where the percentage of infected women has increased 4-fold since 1990. The poor and less educated also appear to be most affected by HIV in Latin America, with more than 60% of all people with AIDS in some regions never having studied beyond primary school. Approximately 1.4 million people in Latin America are currently HIV-positive.

Transmission in the Caribbean continues to be primarily heterosexual. This is reflected in the 5% to 10% rate of seropositivity among pregnant women in Haiti. The overall prevalence of HIV infection in the Caribbean exceeds 2%, making it the second most affected world region after Africa. Approximately 390,000 people in the Caribbean are currently living with HIV infection.

1-5-4 South and Southeast Asia

After Africa, the Asian continent contains the largest population of infected patients, with nearly 7 million HIV-positive people. Although the Asian epidemic was first established in Thailand and has been most studied there, it is growing most rapidly in India and southern China. While the infection seems to have entered these regions through IDU and the commercial sex industry, rates of infection among heterosexuals in many rural areas are increasing rapidly. In some Chinese border states, for example, up to 1% of pregnant women are HIV-positive, and in Tamil Nadu, a state with more than 60 million people in southern India, 5% to 10% of all adults and 25% of single and divorced men living in both rural and urban settings are infected. The most commonly identified risk factors are multiple sex partners, visits to commercial sex workers, and a history of sexually transmitted disease. High rates of infection are also seen in Cambodia, Myanmar, and Vietnam, while in Bangladesh, Indonesia, Laos, Pakistan, the Philippines, and Sri Lanka, infection rates have not yet reached 1 in 1000. The lack of sophisticated systems for diagnosing and treating HIV infections in many countries in South and Southeast Asia, a region that contains nearly half the world's population, augurs poorly for prospects of gaining control of the epidemic in this region in the near future.

1-5-5 Sub-Saharan Africa

The HIV pandemic began in sub-Saharan Africa more than two decades ago, and the region is now home to approximately 70% of the HIV-positive population worldwide, a number estimated to exceed 25 million in December 2000. Sub-Saharan Africa can also lay claim to more than 80% of all AIDS-related deaths, to 9 out of 10 infected children, and to more than 95% of all AIDS orphans; all of this has been inflicted on a region with less than one tenth of the world's population. The southern part of Africa has been particularly hard-hit, including Zimbabwe, Botswana, Namibia, Swaziland, and South Africa. In some regions, more than 25% of all people aged 15 to 49 and up to 50% of pregnant women are infected with HIV. Such high rates of HIV infection have decreased the life expectancy by 5 to 15 years in many African countries.

SELECTED REFERENCES

Ancelle-Park R: Expanded European AIDS case definition. *Lancet* 1993;341:441.

Baltimore D, Heilman C: HIV vaccines: prospects and challenges. *Sci Am* 1998;279:98–103.

Bartlett JG: *The Johns Hopkins Hospital 1998–1999 Guide to Medical Care of Patients With HIV Infection.* 8th ed. Baltimore, MD: Williams & Wilkins; 1999.

Bartlett JG, Moore RD: Improving HIV therapy. *Sci Am* 1998;279:84–87,89.

Belfort R Jr: The ophthalmologist and the global impact of the AIDS epidemic. LV Edward Jackson Memorial Lecture. *Am J Ophthalmol* 2000;129:1–8.

Centers for Disease Control and Prevention: 1993 revised classification system for HIV infection and expanded surveillance case definition for AIDS among adolescents and adults. *MMWR* 1992;41(RR-17):1–19.

Centers for Disease Control and Prevention: Public Health Service guidelines for the management of health-care worker exposures to HIV and recommendations for post-exposure prophylaxis. *MMWR* 1998;47(RR-7):1–33.

Centers for Disease Control and Prevention: The global HIV and AIDS epidemic, 2001. *MMWR* 2001;50:434–439.

Centers for Disease Control and Prevention website on HIV/AIDS prevention: www.cdc.gov/nchstp/hiv_aids/pubs/facts.htm

Coates TJ, Collins C: Preventing HIV infection. *Sci Am* 1998;279:96–97.

Cunningham ET Jr, Margolis TP: Ocular manifestations of HIV infection. *N Engl J Med* 1998;339:236–244.

Eberle J, Habermann J, Gurtler LG: HIV-1 infection transmitted by serum droplets into the eye: a case report. *AIDS* 2000;14:206–207.

Emery S, Lane HC: Immune reconstitution in HIV infection. *Curr Opin Immunol* 1997;9:568–572.

European Centre for the Epidemiological Monitoring of AIDS: 1993 revision of the European AIDS surveillance case definition. *HIV/AIDS Surveillance in Europe.* Quarterly Report. 1993;37:23–28.

European Centre for the Epidemiological Monitoring of AIDS (CESES) website: www.ceses.org

Fahey JL, Flemmig DS, eds: *AIDS/HIV Reference Guide for Medical Professionals.* 4th ed. Baltimore, MD: Williams & Wilkins; 1997.

Fauci AS: The AIDS epidemic: considerations for the 21st century. *N Engl J Med* 1999;341:1046–1050.

Fauci AS, Pantaleo G, Stanley S, et al: Immuno-pathogenic mechanisms of HIV infection. *Ann Intern Med* 1996;124:654–663.

Gayle HD, Hill GL: Global impact of human immunodeficiency virus and AIDS. *Clin Microbiol Rev* 2001;14:327–335.

Grant AD, De Cock KM: The growing challenge of HIV/AIDS in developing countries. *Br Med Bull* 1998;54:369–381.

Greene WC: AIDS and the immune system. *Sci Am* 1993;269:98–105.

JAMA HIV/AIDS Information Center website: www.ama-assn.org/special/hiv/hivhome.htm

Joint United Nations Programme on HIV/AIDS: *AIDS Epidemic Update.* Geneva: UNAIDS; December 2000 and 2001.

Joint United Nations Programme on HIV/AIDS website: www.unaids.org

Jones JL, De Cock KM, Jaffe HW: Current trends in the epidemiology of HIV/AIDS. In: Sande MA, Volberding PA, eds: *The Medical Management of AIDS.* 6th ed. Philadelphia: WB Saunders Co; 1999:3–22.

Jung AC, Paauw DS: Diagnosing HIV-related disease: using the CD4 count as a guide. *J Gen Intern Med* 1998;13:131–136.

Kestelyn PG, Cunningham ET Jr: HIV/AIDS and blindness. *Bull World Health Organ* 2001;79:208–213.

McCune JM: The dynamics of CD4+ T-cell depletion in HIV disease. *Nature* 2001;410:974–979.

McMichael AJ, Rowland-Jones SL: Cellular immune responses to HIV. *Nature* 2001;410:980–987.

Mann JM, Tarantola DJ: HIV 1998: the global picture. *Sci Am* 1998;279:82–83.

Palella FJ Jr, Delaney KM, Moorman AC, et al: Declining morbidity and mortality among patients with advanced human immunodeficiency virus infection. HIV Outpatient Study Investigators. *N Engl J Med* 1998;338:853–860.

Perrin L, Telenti A: HIV treatment failure: testing for HIV resistance in clinical practice. *Science* 1998;280:1871–1873.

Phair JP: Markers and determinants of progression of HIV-1 infection. *J Lab Clin Med* 1998;131:406–409.

Piot P, Bartos M, Ghys PD, et al: The global impact of HIV/AIDS. *Nature* 2001;410:968–973.

Quinn TC: Global burden of the HIV pandemic. *Lancet* 1996;348:99–106.

Satcher D: The global HIV/AIDS epidemic. *JAMA* 1999;281:1479.

Sharp PM, Bailes E, Robertson DL, et al: Origins and evolution of AIDS viruses. *Biol Bull* 1999;196:338–342.

Molecular Mechanisms

Although many aspects of the pathogenesis of HIV infection remain unknown, molecular approaches have elucidated the basic structure and function of the HIV genome and its various gene products. Continued insights into the biology of human HIV infection, including attachment and internalization, reverse transcription of viral RNA, nuclear transport and integration of proviral DNA, transcription and processing of viral RNA, and virion morphogenesis, promise to provide novel targets for future antiretroviral drug development.

Two HIV subtypes infect humans: HIV-1 and HIV-2. While both HIV-1 and HIV-2 are capable of producing AIDS, HIV-1 is by far the more common pathogen. HIV-2 infections, in contrast, are sporadic and limited mostly to isolated regions of West Africa. Only HIV-1 is considered in this chapter.

HIV is now indisputably established as the causative agent of AIDS. The central event in the pathogenesis of AIDS appears to be the preferential infection and depletion of CD4$^+$ T cells. While the mechanisms by which HIV depletes CD4$^+$ cells are undoubtedly complex and multifactorial, demonstration of continued high-level viral replication and of ongoing turnover and replacement of CD4$^+$ lymphocytes throughout the course of infection would seem to suggest a direct cytopathic effect of the virus. This notion is supported by the observation that HIV infection causes CD4$^+$ cell fusion in vitro, thereby forming multinucleated syncytia, a terminal event for infected CD4$^+$ T lymphocytes. Moreover, other HIV-infected cells that fail to form syncytia, such as monocytes and macrophages, are less likely to die following infection. However, some authorities have suggested that HIV infection may also decrease the de novo production of hematopoietic cells. Still other authors have demonstrated that HIV infection is accompanied by apoptosis of both infected and nearby host cells. Ultimately, a complete understanding of HIV-associated pathogenesis will depend on the elucidation of the molecular biology of the virus and of the interaction of HIV with its cellular targets, most notably CD4$^+$ T lymphocytes.

VIRAL GENOME

HIV is a retrovirus of the subfamily Lenti-
virinae. In general, lentivirus infections are
characterized by long periods of clinical latency, by persistent viremia, and by involvement of both the hematopoietic and
the nervous systems. Whereas most retroviruses contain a relatively simple genome,
lentiviruses tend to be more complex. The
RNA genome of HIV is approximately 9
kilobase pairs and contains 9 genes that
produce at least 15 distinct protein products
by way of alternate splicing and/or posttranslational processing. These 15 HIV
gene products include

Four structural proteins:
1. Capsid protein (CA) or p24^{gag}
2. Matrix protein (MA) or p17^{gag}
3. Nucleocapsid protein (NC) or p6^{gag}
4. Nucleocapsid protein (NC) or p7^{gag}

Two envelope proteins:
1. Transmembrane protein (TM) or gp41^{env}
2. Surface protein (SU) or gp120^{env}

Three enzymes:
1. Reverse transcriptase (RT)
2. Integrase (IN)
3. Protease (PR)

Six regulatory proteins:
1. Vpr
2. Nef
3. Vif
4. Tat
5. Rev
6. Vpu

Like all lentiviruses, HIV proviral RNA
is reverse-transcribed to viral DNA by the
viral RT once inside a host cell. HIV proviral DNA is flanked by long terminal repeat
(LTR) sequences, which are important for
transcriptional regulation (Figure 2-1). HIV
structural proteins and enzymes are produced from full-length, unspliced genomic
mRNAs encoded by the *gag* and *pol* genes,
respectively. The envelope proteins and
three of the six regulatory proteins (Vpr,
Vif, and Vpu), in contrast, are generated
from singly spliced subgenomic mRNAs,
while the other three regulatory proteins
(Nef, Tat, and Rev) are produced from
doubly spliced mRNAs.

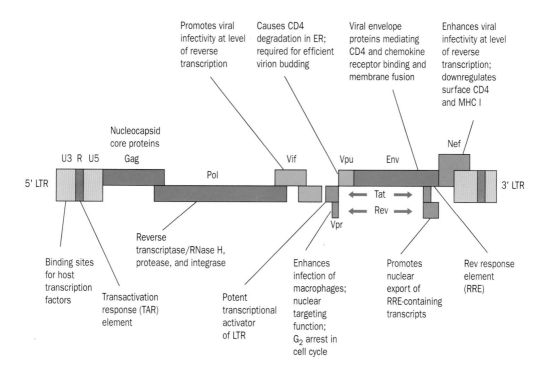

Figure 2-1 *Genomic structure of HIV-1 showing 9 partly overlapping coding regions of the virus. Proposed functions for each gene product are indicated. Subsequent processing of these 9 gene products produces at least 15 distinct proteins in mature virion. LTRs 5' and 3' contain regulatory elements recognized by host transcription factors. HIV-2 genome has very similar structure. ER = endoplasmic reticulum. MHC I = major histocompatibility complex class I.*

Redrawn with permission of the publisher from Geleziunas R, Greene WC: Molecular insights into HIV infection and pathogenesis. In: Sande MA, Volberding PA, eds: The Medical Management of AIDS. *6th ed. Philadelphia: WB Saunders Co; 1999:23–39.*

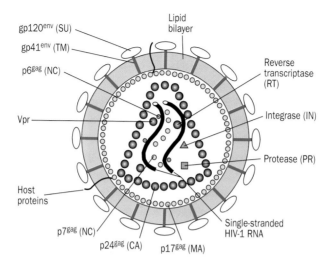

gp120^{env} (SU)

gp41^{env} (TM)

p6^{gag} (NC)

Vpr

Host
proteins

p7^{gag} (NC)

p24^{gag} (CA)   p17^{gag} (MA)

Lipid
bilayer

Reverse
transcriptase
(RT)

Integrase (IN)

Protease (PR)

Single-stranded
HIV-1 RNA

Figure 2-2 *Structure of HIV-1 virion. Proteins comprising virus envelope (TM or gp41^{env} and SU or gp120^{env}) and inner core (NC or p7^{gag}, NC or p6^{gag}, CA or p24^{gag}, MA or p17^{gag}) are identified, as are diploid RNA genome, reverse transcriptase (RT), integrase (IN), protease (PR), Vpr, lipid bilayer, and host proteins. Nef and Vif are also found in virion, but are not shown. TM = transmembrane protein. SU = surface protein. NC = nucleocapsid protein. CA = capsid protein. MA = matrix protein.*
Redrawn with permission of the publisher from Gelez"zunas R, Greene WC: Molecular insights into HIV infection and pathogenesis. In: Sande MA, Volberding PA, eds: The Medical Management of AIDS. 6th ed. Philadelphia: WB Saunders Co; 1999:23–39.

2-2

VIRION STRUCTURE

The HIV virion is a complex structure composed of concentric, overlapping layers (Figure 2-2). The retroviral core contains two copies of single-stranded HIV genomic RNA in close association with two HIV-encoded RNA-binding NC proteins (p6^{gag} and p7^{gag}). The three HIV-encoded enzymes (RT, IN, and PR), as well as the regulatory proteins Vpr, Nef, and Vif, are also in the retroviral core. The core is covered, in turn, by a conical shell of CA protein (p24^{gag}), which itself is surrounded by MA protein (p17^{gag}). NC proteins, MA, and CA are each proteolytically cleaved from p60 Gag precursor by HIV protease. A lipid bilayer, which contains the two major virus envelope proteins (TM or gp41^{env} and SU or gp120^{env}), surrounds the inner conical structure. The lipid bilayer also contains numerous host proteins, including class I and class II major histocompatibility complex (MHC) antigens, actin, and ubiquitin, which are acquired during virion budding.

CELLULAR ATTACHMENT AND ENTRY

HIV enters target cells by attaching via the envelope glycoprotein gp120^{env} to the CD4 receptor, expressed primarily on lymphocytes, monocytes, and macrophages. Although the gp120–CD4 receptor interaction is high-affinity, it alone is insufficient to mediate HIV entry, which requires the presence of one or more coreceptors. These HIV coreceptors are now known to be members of a family of seven transmembrane G-protein–coupled receptors, the natural ligands for which are chemokines. Entry can be competitively blocked by the natural ligands of these receptors. The best-characterized of the HIV chemokine coreceptors are CCR5 and CXCR4, which are important for binding of HIV to macrophages and T lymphocytes, respectively. Chemokine receptor utilization preference appears to determine differences in HIV tropism, a phenomenon that appears to reside in a hypervariable region of the gp120^{env} protein termed V3. Evidence suggests that HIV chemokine receptor preferences can change during the course of HIV infection, due primarily to continual changes in the V3 region. Nonhematopoietic cells may also be infected by HIV, including microglial cells in the brain and epithelial cells in the gastrointestinal tract.

Fusion of HIV with the target cells is mediated by the gp41^{env} protein, which appears to anchor both itself and gp120^{env} in the lipid bilayer of the virus. Once gp120^{env} recognizes the CD4 receptor and its V3 region binds to a cognate chemokine receptor, the amino terminal portion of gp41^{env} undergoes a conformational change to activate fusion, thus enabling the viral and host cell membranes to fuse (Figure 2-3).

VIRAL REVERSE TRANSCRIPTION AND DNA INTEGRATION

Once entry of HIV into the host cell has been completed, the virion coat is removed and viral RT generates double-stranded DNA copies from each single-stranded viral RNA genome. Two HIV regulatory proteins that are also in the virion, Nef and Vif, appear to enhance the reverse-transcription process. The double-stranded DNA replica of the original HIV RNA genome is then imported into the nucleus of the infected cell and integrated into the host DNA by the viral enzyme integrase. The process of nuclear importation of HIV is incompletely understood, but it is generally believed that at least three HIV proteins assist in this process: Vpr, matrix, and integrase. Vpr also causes cells to arrest in the G$_2$ phase of the cell cycle.

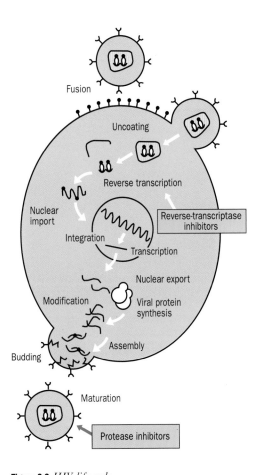

Figure 2-3 *HIV life cycle.*

Modified with permission from Trono D: Molecular biology and the development of AIDS therapeutics. AIDS *1996;10 (suppl 3):S53-S59. Copyright © 1996 Lippincott Williams & Williams.*

2-5

VIRAL LATENCY

Clinically, HIV "latency" is something of a misnomer. In fact, within several months of infection, patients produce a relatively stable level of between 10^3 and 10^6 copies of HIV RNA per milliliter of plasma, and HIV-infected T cells die and are replaced every couple of days. The exact level of circulating HIV particles is determined by host genetics and the virulence of a given virus isolate. Each mature virion has a serum half-life of less than 6 hours.

HIV infection of any given CD4+ T lymphocyte may be either productive or latent. Productive HIV replication generally requires T-cell activation, for example, by antigens, mitogens, pro-inflammatory cytokines such as interleukin-1 or tumor necrosis factor, or by coinfection by other viruses such as herpes simplex virus (HSV) or cytomegalovirus (CMV). Resting T cells, in contrast, cannot support HIV replication. Because memory T cells have the longest life span of any CD4+ lymphocytic subset (at least 6 months), they represent the greatest cellular reservoir of latent HIV. T-cell activation usually stimulates the potent transcription factor NF-κB, multiple binding sites for which are present in the HIV proviral LTR.

2-6

VIRAL REGULATORY AND STRUCTURAL GENES

Three HIV regulatory proteins are produced soon after T-cell activation: Tat, Rev, and Nef. Tat protein is a potent HIV transactivator and is essential for HIV replication. Tat binds both to the 5′ end of nascent HIV transcripts, thereby enhancing transcriptional elongation of these mRNAs. Tat function appears to require the presence of a cellular factor encoded on chromosome 12, cyclin T. Rev protein, like Tat protein, is critical for HIV replication. The main function of Rev appears to be enhancing the nuclear export of unspliced and singly spliced HIV structural, enzymatic, and regulatory gene transcripts that encode proteins required for virion assembly. Nef protein appears to have multiple roles. In addition to the facilitative effect Nef has on reverse transcription, Nef causes CD4 receptor and MHC I downregulation. CD4 receptor downregulation may facilitate budding of viral particles, possibly by preventing attachment to the host cell during egress.

2-7

VIRION ASSEMBLY

HIV gene products are cleaved by the concerted action of both host and viral proteases to produce the final proteins that are present in the virion. Virion assembly starts with aggregation of the ribonucleotide cores beneath the plasma membrane. HIV cores are composed of viral RNA, the various posttranslationally processed Gag proteins, and the enzymes variably transcribed from the *pol* gene. Budding then proceeds, incorporating both HIV envelope proteins and host membrane components into the virion lipid bilayer. Once budding is complete, HIV protease is activated and finalizes the maturation of the virion. Like Nef protein, Vpu appears to enhance HIV production by downregulating surface expression of CD4 receptors, thereby minimizing the chance for surface CD4 receptors to slow the shedding process. Vif appears to act to enhance proviral DNA synthesis.

2-8

ANTIRETROVIRAL AGENTS

Three broad classes of antiretroviral agents are in clinical use: nucleoside analogs, protease inhibitors, and nonnucleoside reverse-transcriptase inhibitors.

Nucleoside analogs preferentially inhibit reverse transcription of HIV genomic RNA into double-stranded proviral DNA. Six nucleoside analogs are currently available (trade names are in parentheses following the generic names):

1. Zidovudine (ZDV, AZT, Retrovir)
2. Didanosine (ddI, Videx)
3. Zalcitabine (ddC, HIVID)
4. Stavudine (d4T, Zerit)
5. Lamivudine (3TC, Epivir)
6. Abacavir (ABC, Ziagen)

Protease inhibitors, in contrast, inhibit the HIV enzyme protease (PR), which is required for posttranslational processing of HIV structural proteins. Protease inhibitors are generally more potent than nucleoside analogs as inhibitors of HIV replication. Six protease inhibitors are currently available:

1. Amprenavir (Agenerase)
2. Indinavir (Crixivan)
3. Nelfinavir (Viracept)
4. Ritonavir (Norvir)
5. Saquinavir (Fortovase)
6. Lipinovir, which is available in combination with ritonavir (Kaletra)

Nonnucleoside reverse-transcriptase inhibitors (NNRTI) inhibit the HIV enzyme reverse transcriptase (RT) by binding adjacent to the active site of the enzyme, causing a conformational change in the molecule. Three NNRTIs are currently available:

1. Nevirapine (Viramune)
2. Delavirdine (Rescriptor)
3. Efavirenz (Sustiva)

The combined use of three or four of these antiretroviral agents is referred to as *highly active antiretroviral therapy* (HAART), and only by using three or more drugs in combination is the potency sufficient to generate sustained suppression without the outgrowth of resistant virus. Therapy usually begins with a combination of two nucleoside analogs and either a protease inhibitor or an NNRTI. The choice of agents in any given patient is complex and depends on an assessment of combined drug potency, expected duration of benefit, prior drug resistance and toxicity profiles, potential interactions with other medications, convenience of dosing, and cost. While adequate viral suppression is achieved in most patients, a sizable proportion of patients fail to achieve the desired level of viral suppression due to problems with adherence, drug interactions, and toxicity.

SELECTED REFERENCES

Cairns JS, D'Souza MP: Chemokines and HIV-1 second receptors: the therapeutic connection. *Nat Med* 1998;4:563–568.

Carpenter CC, Cooper DA, Fischl MA, et al: Antiretroviral therapy in adults: updated recommendations of the International AIDS Society–USA Panel. *JAMA* 2000;283:381–390.

Chan DC, Kim PS: HIV entry and its inhibition. *Cell* 1998;93:681–684.

Cohen OJ, Kinter A, Fauci AS: Host factors in the pathogenesis of HIV disease. *Immunol Rev* 1997;159:31–48.

Cullen BR: HIV-1 auxiliary proteins: making connections in a dying cell. *Cell* 1998;93:685–692.

Deeks SG, Volberding PA: Antiretroviral therapy. In: Sande MA, Volberding PA, eds: *The Medical Management of AIDS.* 6th ed. Philadelphia: WB Saunders Co; 1999:97–115.

D'Souza MP, Cairns JS, Plaeger SF: Current evidence and future directions for targeting HIV entry: therapeutic and prophylactic strategies. *JAMA* 2000;284: 215–222.

Fauci AS: Host factors and the pathogenesis of HIV-induced disease. *Nature* 1996;384:529–534.

Finzi D, Siliciano RF: Viral dynamics in HIV-1 infection. *Cell* 1998;93:665–671.

Geleziunas R, Greene WC: Molecular insights into HIV infection and pathogenesis. In: Sande MA, Volberding PA, eds: *The Medical Management of AIDS.* 6th ed. Philadelphia: WB Saunders Co; 1999:23–39.

Graziosi C, Soudeyns H, Rizzardi GP, et al: Immunopathogenesis of HIV infection. *AIDS Res Hum Retroviruses* 1998;14(suppl 2):S135–S142.

Greene WC: The molecular biology of human immunodeficiency virus type 1 infection. *N Engl J Med* 1991;324:308–317.

Levy JA, Kaminsky LS, Morrow WJ, et al: Infection by the retrovirus associated with the acquired immunodeficiency syndrome: clinical, biological, and molecular features. *Ann Intern Med* 1985;103:694–699.

Littman DR: Chemokine receptors: keys to AIDS pathogenesis? *Cell* 1998;93:677–680.

McCune JM: The dynamics of CD4+ T-cell depletion in HIV disease. *Nature* 2001:410: 974–979.

McMichael A: T cell responses and viral escape. *Cell* 1998;93:673–676.

McMichael AJ, Rowland-Jones SL: Cellular immune responses to HIV. *Nature* 2001;410: 980–987.

Richman DD: HIV chemotherapy. *Nature* 2001; 410:995–1001.

Strebel K, Bour S: Molecular interactions of HIV with host factors. *AIDS* 1999;13(suppl A): S13–S24.

Trono D: Molecular biology and the development of AIDS therapeutics. *AIDS* 1996;10 (suppl 3):S53–S59.

Turner BG, Summers MF: Structural biology of HIV. *J Mol Biol* 1999;285:1–32.

CHAPTER 3

Prevention of HIV Transmission

All body fluids may potentially transmit disease, including HIV infection. Health care workers who care for HIV-infected patients should therefore take appropriate measures to minimize the risk of transmission, both to themselves and between patients.

3-1

UNIVERSAL PRECAUTIONS

Universal precautions have been developed to minimize the risk of infection of health care workers who are exposed to potentially infectious body fluids. These precautions include appropriate use of protective barriers, hand-washing, and disposal of needles and other sharp instruments ("sharps"). The Centers for Disease Control and Prevention (CDC) has recommended the following precautions:

1. All health care workers should routinely use appropriate barrier precautions to prevent skin and mucous membrane exposure when in contact with blood, body fluids containing visible blood, and other body fluids to which universal precautions apply, such as semen, vaginal secretions, cerebrospinal fluid, synovial fluid, pleural fluid, peritoneal fluid, pericardial fluid, and amniotic fluid. Gloves should be worn for touching blood and body fluids, mucous membranes, or nonintact skin of all patients, for handling items or surfaces soiled with blood or body fluids, and for performing venipuncture and other vascular access procedures. Gloves should be discarded properly after contact with each patient. To prevent exposure of mucous membranes of the mouth, nose, and eyes, a mask and protective eyewear or a face shield should be worn during procedures that are likely to generate droplets of blood or other body fluids. A gown or an apron should be worn during procedures that are likely to generate splashes of blood or other body fluids.

2. Hands and other skin surfaces should be washed immediately and thoroughly if contaminated with blood, body fluids containing visible blood, and other body fluids to which universal precautions apply. Hands should be washed immediately after gloves are removed.

3. All health care workers should take precautions to prevent injuries caused by needles, scalpels, and other sharp instruments or devices during procedures, when cleaning used instruments, during disposal of used needles, and when handling sharp instruments after procedures. To prevent needle-stick injuries, needles should not be recapped, not purposely bent or broken by hand, not removed from disposable syringes, nor otherwise manipulated by hand.

After use, disposable syringes and needles, scalpel blades, and other sharp items should be placed in puncture-resistant containers to be used for disposal. The puncture-resistant containers should be located as close as is practical to the use area, preferably in each patient room. Large-bore reusable needles should be placed in a puncture-resistant container for transport to the reprocessing area.

4. There has been one possible case in which saliva has been implicated in HIV transmission. Therefore, the need for emergency mouth-to-mouth resuscitation should be minimized. Mouthpieces, resuscitation bags, or other ventilation devices should be available for use in areas in which the need for resuscitation is predictable. Disposable airway equipment and devices should be used. Such equipment should be used only once and then disposed of properly.

5. Health care workers who have exudative lesions or weeping dermatitis should refrain from all direct patient care and from handling patient care equipment until the condition resolves.

6. Pregnant health care workers are not known to be at greater risk of contracting HIV infection than nonpregnant health care workers. However, if a health care worker develops HIV infection during or prior to pregnancy, the infant is at risk of infection from perinatal transmission. Pregnant health care workers should, therefore, be especially familiar with, and strictly adhere to, precautions to minimize the risk of HIV transmission.

7. Isolation precautions should be taken as necessary if associated conditions, such as infectious diarrhea or tuberculosis, are diagnosed or suspected.

Some body fluids and excretions are associated with a very low risk of HIV transmission, including feces, nasal secretions, sputum, sweat, urine, vomitus, tears, aqueous humor, and vitreous. Transmission remains possible, however, particularly when these fluids contain visible blood, so prudent precautions should be taken.

3-2

OSHA STANDARDS

The Occupational Safety and Health Administration (OSHA) standards on exposure to blood-borne pathogens have been in effect in the United States since March of 1992. These standards outline safeguards that employers must provide for their employees to protect them against occupational exposures. OSHA standards restate and extend the CDC recommendations listed above. In brief, employers should

1. Identify tasks that present a risk of exposure, as well as identify those employees who will be performing those tasks

2. Provide both methods and schedules for implementing protective barriers, safe workplace practices, and engineering controls to reduce the risk of exposure

3. Outline requirements for general housekeeping, cleaning and disinfection, handling and disposal of infectious waste and sharps, and management of soiled linen

4. Provide hepatitis B vaccinations to employees who are frequently exposed to blood and other potentially infectious materials

5. Provide postexposure evaluations and medical followup

6. Communicate hazards and risks with warning signs and labels

7. Meet special requirements for research laboratories and production facilities

8. Train employees to handle hazards and risks

9. Keep complete safety records

OSHA has complete authority to inspect health care facilities to ensure that its guidelines are fully implemented in the United States.

3-3

TRANSMISSION TO EYE CARE PROFESSIONALS

There has been no documented case of HIV transmission to an eye care professional. Nonetheless, universal precautions, as well as the following special precautions, have been recommended by the CDC for all health care professionals who care for HIV-infected eye patients:

1. Eye care professionals performing eye examinations or procedures involving contact with tears or other body fluids should wash their hands immediately after an examination or procedure and between pa-

tients. Although hand-washing alone should be sufficient, disposable gloves may be worn when practical and convenient. The use of gloves is advised when there are cuts, scratches, or dermatologic lesions on the hands. Protective wear, such as masks, goggles, and gowns, is not indicated.

2. Instruments that contact the eye or tears, such as tonometry tips, should be wiped clean and then disinfected by a 5- to 50-minute exposure to one of the following solutions: (**a**) a fresh solution of 3% hydrogen peroxide; (**b**) a 1/10 dilution of sodium hypochlorite (common household bleach) in 70% ethanol or 70% isopropanol. The instrument should be thoroughly rinsed in tap water and dried before being used again.

3. Trial contact lenses should be disinfected after each fitting with one of the following regimens: (**a**) Hard lenses can be disinfected with a commercially available hydrogen peroxide contact-lens disinfecting system that is currently approved for soft contact lenses. Most hard trial-fitting lenses can also be treated with the standard heat disinfection regimen used for soft lenses, specifically 70°C to 80°C (172°F to 176°F) for 10 minutes. Suppliers of hard contact lenses can be contacted to determine which trial lenses can be safely treated. (**b**) Rigid gas-permeable trial-fitting lenses can be disinfected using the hydrogen peroxide disinfection system described above. Heat disinfection should not be used, as it can warp rigid lenses. (**c**) Soft trial-fitting lenses can be disinfected using the hydrogen peroxide system described above. Some soft lenses can be heat-disinfected. Most standard chemical disinfectants have not been tested for their ability to kill HIV.

3-3-1 Office Transmission

Although HIV has been isolated from tears, from most ocular tissues, and from both contact lenses and their cases, levels are low and these sources are not thought to represent a high risk for transmission. In fact, transmission of HIV from a patient to an eye care professional has not been documented. Nonetheless, the CDC and OSHA standards should be followed in every eye care professional's office. In addition, the Academy has made the following additional recommendations to cover this special circumstance:

1. The tips of eyedrop bottles should not come into direct contact with the ocular surface.

2. Goldmann tonometer tips should be disinfected between patients for 5 minutes with either 1/10 sodium hypochlorite (common household bleach) or 3% hydrogen peroxide. Alternatively, the tips can be thoroughly cleaned with isopropyl alcohol on a sponge. All tips should be rinsed completely and dried after cleaning.

3. Schiotz tonometers should be disinfected between patients. Cleaning can be performed by disassembling the tonometer. The pad can then be cleaned with an alcohol swab, and the barrel with an alcohol-soaked pipe cleaner. The Schiotz tonometer should be rinsed completely and dried after cleaning.

4. Gloves should be worn during venipuncture performed for fluorescein or indocyanine green angiography.

3-3-2 Operating Room Transmission

The surgical setting presents special risks for the transmission of blood-borne pathogens because of the highly invasive nature of the procedures performed and the continuous handling of needles, scalpels, and other sharp instruments. While universal precautions and OSHA standards should be followed during all surgical procedures, the following additional points should be considered when surgery is performed on HIV-positive patients:

1. Needles and sharp instruments should not be recapped, and especially not by the two-handed technique.

2. The "hands-free" or "no-touch" technique should be used to pass needles and sharp instruments. This means that the surgeon, assistant, and scrub nurse do not handle an instrument at the same time. A neutral area, such as a clean instrument table or basin, may be used to transfer instruments.

3. Corneal and scleral donor tissue should be screened for HIV prior to use.

4. Double gloving should be considered, as this may decrease the risk of transmission following percutaneous exposure.

SELECTED REFERENCES

Ablashi DV, Sturzenegger S, Hunter EA, et al: Presence of HTLV-III in tears and cells from the eyes of AIDS patients. *J Exp Pathol* 1987;3: 693–703.

Amin RM, Dean MT, Zaumetzer LE, et al: Virucidal efficacy of various lens cleaning and disinfecting solutions on HIV-I contaminated contact lenses. *AIDS Res Hum Retroviruses* 1991; 7:403–408.

Cantrill HL, Henry K, Jackson B, et al: Recovery of human immunodeficiency virus from ocular tissues in patients with acquired immune deficiency syndrome. *Ophthalmology* 1988;95: 1458–1462.

Centers for Disease Control and Prevention: Guidelines for the prevention of transmission of human immunodeficiency virus, hepatitis B virus, and other bloodborne pathogens in healthcare settings. *MMWR* 1988;37:377–382, 387–388.

Centers for Disease Control and Prevention: Recommendations for preventing possible transmission of human T-lymphotropic virus type III/lymphadenopathy-associated virus from tears. *MMWR* 1985;34:533–534.

Centers for Disease Control and Prevention: Recommendations for prevention of HIV transmission in health-care settings. *MMWR* 1987;36 (suppl 2):1S–18S.

Crutcher JM, Lamm SH, Hall TA: Procedures to protect health-care workers from HIV infection: category I (health-care) workers. *Am Ind Hyg Assoc J* 1991;52:A100–A103.

Driebe WT Jr, Slonim CB: Prevention of HIV transmission in the office and operating room. In: Stenson SM, Friedberg DN, eds: *AIDS and the Eye*. New Orleans: Contact Lens Association of Ophthalmologists; 1995:23–34.

Fahey JL, Flemmig DS, eds: *AIDS/HIV Reference Guide for Medical Professionals*. 4th ed. Baltimore, MD: Williams & Wilkins; 1997.

Fujikawa LS, Salahuddin SZ, Ablashi D, et al: HTLV-III in the tears of AIDS patients. *Ophthalmology* 1986;93:1479–1481.

Ippolito G, Puro V, De Carli G: The risk of occupational human immunodeficiency virus infection in health care workers. Italian Multicenter Study. The Italian Study Group on Occupational Risk of HIV Infection. *Arch Intern Med* 1993;153: 1451–1458.

Marcus R: Surveillance of health care workers exposed to blood from patients infected with the human immunodeficiency virus. *N Engl J Med* 1988;319:1118–1123.

Pepose JS: Contact lens disinfection to prevent transmission of viral disease. *CLAO J* 1988;14: 165–168.

Pepose JS, Linette G, Lee SF, et al: Disinfection of Goldmann tonometers against human immunodeficiency virus type 1. *Arch Ophthalmol* 1989; 107:983–985.

Pugliese G, Lynch P, Jackson M: *Universal Precautions: Policies, Procedures, and Resources*. Chicago: American Hospital Publishing, Inc; 1991.

Tervo T, Lahdevirta J, Vaheri A, et al: Recovery of HTLV-III from contact lenses. *Lancet* 1986;1: 379–380.

Updated Recommendations for Ophthalmic Practice in Relation to the Human Immunodeficiency Virus and Other Infectious Agents. Information Statement. San Francisco: American Academy of Ophthalmology; 1992.

Vogt MW, Ho DD, Bakar SR, et al: Safe disinfection of contact lenses after contamination with HTLV-III. *Ophthalmology* 1986;93:771–774.

CHAPTER 4

Adnexal and Orbital Manifestations

As with all manifestations of HIV infection, adnexal and orbital complications have become far less common in the developed world since the advent of highly active antiretroviral therapy (HAART). Adnexal and orbital complications still affect more than 25% of untreated HIV-positive patients, however, and may be the presenting sign of disease.

4-1

ADNEXAL MANIFESTATIONS

The ocular adnexa include the eyelids, eyelashes, conjunctiva, and lacrimal drainage system. Each of these structures may be involved individually or together by opportunistic infectious or neoplastic disorders associated with HIV infection.

4-1-1 Herpes Zoster Ophthalmicus

Herpes zoster ophthalmicus (HZO) refers to a varicella zoster virus (VZV)–related vesiculobullous dermatitis involving the ophthalmic distribution of the trigeminal nerve (Figure 4-1). HZO affects about 5% to 15% of untreated HIV-infected patients in the developed world and appears to be even more common in Africa. While VZV dermatitis may occur in otherwise normal elderly patients, its occurrence in someone under 50 years of age is uncommon and should raise the suspicion of systemic immunosuppression due to malig-

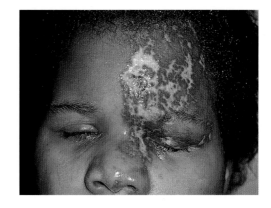

Figure 4-1 *Herpes zoster ophthalmicus.*

nancy, pharmacologic immunosuppression, or HIV infection. This appears to be particularly true in sub-Saharan Africa, where more than 90% of patients who present with HZO are found to be HIV-positive.

While HZO may develop at any CD4+ cell count, it occurs more commonly at CD4+ T-lymphocyte counts less than 200 cells/µL. VZV infections are considered to be disseminated if they involve multiple dermatomes or unrelated organ systems. Ocular complications of HZO occur in approximately 50% of HIV-infected patients and can include keratitis, scleritis, uveitis, retinitis, and optic neuritis.

Standard treatment of HZO involves acyclovir, which is a guanosine analog that is activated via phosphorylation by a virus-specific thymidine kinase. Phosphorylated acyclovir acts to preferentially inhibit viral DNA polymerase, thereby causing DNA chain termination. Initial therapy for HIV-positive patients includes a 1-week course of acyclovir given intravenously at a dose of 10 mg/kg every 8 hours. This treatment is then followed by oral maintenance therapy at 800 mg 5 times daily.

Famciclovir, the diacetyl ester of 6-deoxy-penciclovir, is similar in structure to acyclovir and was approved by the Federal Drug Administration (FDA) for the treatment of herpes zoster infections in 1994. Famciclovir offers the advantage over acyclovir of decreased dosing at 500 mg 3 times daily and appears to be as effective as acyclovir at preventing ocular complications of HZO.

For patients initially unresponsive to acyclovir or for those who show reactivation while taking oral acyclovir or famciclovir, a trial of intravenous foscarnet should be considered. Valacyclovir has been associated with isolated reports of thrombocytopenic purpuric/hemolytic uremic syndrome in profoundly immunosuppressed HIV-positive patients and should, therefore, be used with caution in these patients.

4-1-2 Kaposi Sarcoma

Kaposi sarcoma is a highly vascularized mesenchymal tumor of the skin and mucous membranes caused by human herpes virus-8 infection. Kaposi sarcoma is the most frequently encountered AIDS-related malignancy, occurring in up to 25% of untreated HIV-positive patients. Approximately 5% of untreated patients infected with HIV develop Kaposi sarcoma involving the ocular adnexa. Both the eyelids and the conjunctiva may be involved. Lesions can be of the upper or lower eyelids, or both (Figure 4-2). Extensive lesions can severely compromise lid function and limit vision. Small lesions, in contrast, infrequently affect vision, but can be cosmetically unacceptable to the patient. Conjunctival lesions may occur on any aspect of the palpebral or bulbar conjunctiva and are often mistaken for subconjunctival hemorrhage (Figures 4-3 and 4-4). Bacillary angiomatosis involving the conjunctiva may mimic Kaposi sarcoma and should be considered in any HIV-positive patient with a history of systemic *Bartonella* infection or cat-scratch disease.

Patients often request treatment of adnexal Kaposi sarcoma for cosmetic reasons. In addition, therapy may be indicated to

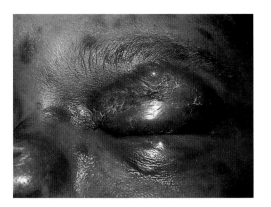

Figure **4-2** *Extensive Kaposi sarcoma of face and eyelids, limiting vision.*

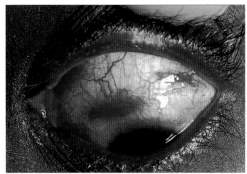

A

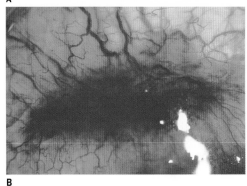

B

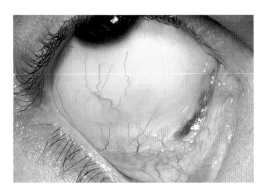

Figure **4-3** *Kaposi sarcoma in inferior cul-de-sac, mimicking subconjunctival hemorrhage.*

Figure **4-4** *(A) Multiple Kaposi sarcoma lesions on bulbar conjunctiva. (B) High-power view of one such lesion reveals its vascular nature.*

prevent or reverse complications such as entropion, ectropion, trichiasis, epiphora, exposure, or obstruction of vision. Radiation therapy is effective at treating eyelid and conjunctival Kaposi sarcoma, but radiation is expensive and can be associated with loss of lashes, skin irritation, and conjunctivitis. Isolated lesions of the eyelid may also be treated by cryotherapy or with intralesional vinblastine or interferon alpha.

Excision can be performed, but is often difficult and tends to be complicated by bleeding. Conjunctival lesions also respond to cryotherapy or intralesional chemotherapy, but, unlike eyelid lesions, can be excised with relative ease. Fluorescein angiography of the anterior segment is occasionally helpful to identify a tumor-free margin of 1 to 2 mm at the time of surgery. Eyelid or conjunctival lesions accompanied by systemic involvement are usually best treated with systemic chemotherapy, such as liposomal daunorubicin or doxorubicin. Recurrences of Kaposi sarcoma are common as long as immune suppression continues. Successful HAART may produce spontaneous and sustained remission of Kaposi sarcoma such that treatment can often be foregone while HAART is initiated to allow the immune system to reconstitute.

4-1-3 Molluscum Contagiosum

Molluscum contagiosum is a highly contagious papulonodular dermatitis caused by a DNA poxvirus. Both the skin and the mucous membranes may be affected, typically with multiple small umbilicated lesions. Molluscum contagiosum is more common in patients infected with HIV and, when present, tends to be more severe, with larger, more numerous, and more rapidly growing lesions. The face, trunk, and genitalia are the most common sites of involvement. Occurrence on the eyelids affects less than 5% of patients (Figure 4-5). Conjunctival molluscum contagiosum has been described, but is extremely uncommon. Associated follicular conjunctivitis and superficial keratitis frequently occur in immunocompetent patients, but appear to be less common in HIV-infected individuals. Treatment options include cryotherapy, excision and curettage, or simple incision of the dome of the lesions.

4-1-4 Squamous Cell Carcinoma

Patients infected with HIV appear to be at increased risk for developing conjunctival and eyelid squamous cell carcinoma, or conjunctival intraepithelial neoplasms (Figure 4-6). The condition is believed to be associated with human papillomavirus (HPV) infection. Such tumors have been reported in HIV-positive patients in Africa and Brazil, but are relatively uncommon. Diagnosis and treatment involve wide excisional biopsy with frozen-section monitoring of the margins and cryotherapy applied to the edges. A single case of basal cell carcinoma has been reported in a patient with AIDS.

4-1-5 Cutaneous Lymphoma

Non-Hodgkin lymphoma is more common, and tends to be of higher-grade malignancy, in patients infected with HIV than in noninfected patients. A patient with non-Hodgkin lymphoma of the eyelid has been described, but such lesions appear to be quite rare. Conjunctival lymphoma usually responds to local radiation therapy.

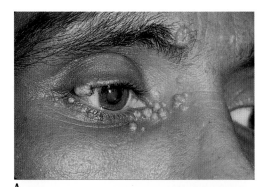

A

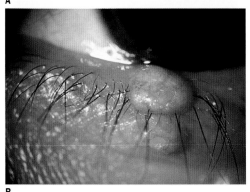

B

Figure 4-5 *(A) Multiple periocular molluscum conta-giosum lesions. (B) High-power view of two mollus-cum contagiosum lesions on inferior lid margin.*

Part A reproduced with permission from Cunningham ET Jr, Margolis TP: Ocular manifestations of HIV infection. N Engl J Med 1998;339:236-244. Copyright © 1998 Massachusetts Medical Society. All rights reserved. Part B courtesy Cristina Muccioli, MD.

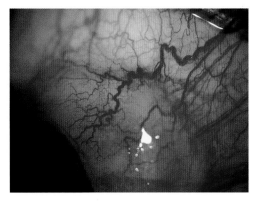

Figure 4-6 *Squamous cell carcinoma of conjunctiva at superior limbus.*

Courtesy Cristina Muccioli, MD.

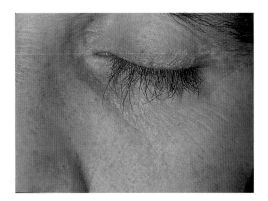

Figure 4-7 *Trichomegaly, or excessively long eyelashes.*

4-1-6 Trichomegaly

Acquired trichomegaly, or hypertrichosis of the eyelashes, typically occurs in the late stages of HIV infection (Figure 4-7). The cause of trichomegaly is unknown, although elevated viral titers, drug toxicity, and poor nutrition have all been suggested as con-tributing factors. Excessively long lashes

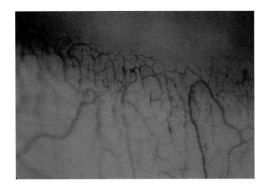

Figure 4-8 *Conjunctival microvascular changes at inferior limbus.*

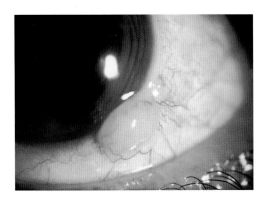

Figure 4-9 *Conjunctival* Cryptococcus *in setting of disseminated disease.*
Courtesy Cristina Muccioli, MD.

may be trimmed as needed if they interfere with the use of spectacles or if they are cosmetically unacceptable to the patient.

4-1-7 Conjunctival Microvasculopathy

Conjunctival microvascular changes are said to be common in severely immunosuppressed HIV-positive patients. Typical findings include segmental vascular dilation and narrowing, microaneurysm formation, the appearance of comma-shaped vascular fragments, and a visible granularity to the flowing blood column, termed *sludging.* These changes are usually most evident near the limbus inferiorly (Figure 4-8) and are highly correlated with the occurrence of retinal microvasculopathy, both of which are most common at CD4$^+$ T-lymphocyte counts less than 100 cells/μL.

The reason for the occurrence of conjunctival microvascular changes in the setting of HIV infection is unknown. Theories have included an HIV-induced increase in plasma viscosity (perhaps related to increased blood cell rigidity), HIV-related immune-complex deposition, and direct infection of the conjunctival vascular endothelium by HIV. No treatment is required for this condition.

4-1-8 Conjunctivitis

The prevalence of conjunctivitis in patients with AIDS is similar to that in the general population. Uncommon infectious forms of conjunctivitis that have been reported in patients infected by HIV, however, include cytomegalovirus (CMV) conjunctivitis and cryptococcal conjunctivitis (Figure 4-9). Treatment of suspected conjunctivitis should be guided by the results of Gram stains and cultures.

4-1-9 Preseptal Cellulitis

Preseptal cellulitis caused by *Staphylococcus aureus* has been described in a number of HIV-positive patients. This is perhaps not unexpected since HIV-infected patients carry *S aureus* in their nares nearly twice as often as normal controls. In fact, *S aureus* appears to be the most common cause of cutaneous and systemic bacterial infections in patients with AIDS. The infection usually responds promptly to oral therapy with penicillinase-resistant penicillin, such as methicillin, which should be continued for 10 days. Failure to respond to therapy should prompt hospitalization for a computed tomography (CT) or magnetic resonance imaging (MRI) study of the orbit to rule out sinusitis and for intravenous antibiotic therapy.

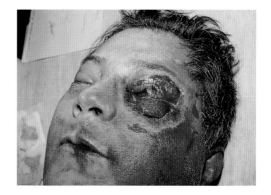

Figure 4-10 *Fatal orbital cellulitis due to* Staphylococcus aureus.
Courtesy Cristina Muccioli, MD.

4-2

ORBITAL MANIFESTATIONS

Orbital manifestations of HIV are relatively uncommon, affecting less than 1% of patients. Such complications may be serious, however, and deserve prompt medical attention. Symptoms often include pain, decreased vision, or diplopia. Frequent signs include ptosis, proptosis, erythema, chemosis, limited extraocular motility, decreased vision, elevated intraocular pressure, and an afferent pupillary defect.

The most common orbital complications in patients with AIDS are orbital cellulitis (Figure 4-10) and non-Hodgkin lymphoma (Figure 4-11). Among HIV-infected patients with orbital cellulitis, *Aspergillus* species are the most commonly identified organisms, although patients with orbital cellulitis

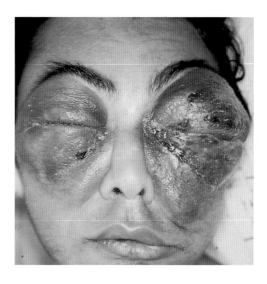

Figure 4-11 *Bilateral lid swelling due to orbital lymphoma.*
Courtesy Cristina Muccioli, MD.

caused by *Propionibacterium acnes, Pseudomonas aeruginosa, Staphylococcus aureus, Treponema pallidum, Rhizopus arrhizus, Toxoplasma gondii,* and *Pneumocystis carinii* have also been reported. Concurrent infection of one or more of the sinuses and intracranial extension are common. Therapy for orbital cellulitis includes systemic antibiotics and, as indicated, surgical debridement.

Isolated reports of orbital Kaposi sarcoma, inflammatory pseudotumor, orbital myositis, orbital eosinophilic granuloma, and metastatic carcinoma to the orbit have also been described. Diagnosis requires orbital CT or MRI followed by biopsy and/or culture, as indicated. Lymphoma and Kaposi sarcoma are treated with radiation and chemotherapy, respectively.

SELECTED REFERENCES

Acharya NR, Cunningham ET Jr: Corneal, anterior segment, and adnexal manifestations of human immunodeficiency virus. *Int Ophthalmol Clin* 1998;38:161–177.

Akduman L, Pepose JS: Anterior segment manifestations of acquired immunodeficiency syndrome. *Sem Ophthalmol* 1995;10:111–118.

Ateenyi-Agaba C: Conjunctival squamous-cell carcinoma associated with HIV infection in Kampala, Uganda. *Lancet* 1995;345:695–696.

Bardenstein DS, Elmets C: Hyperfocal cryotherapy of multiple molluscum contagiosum lesions in patients with the acquired immune deficiency syndrome. *Ophthalmology* 1995;102:1031–1034.

Colin J, Prisant O, Cochener B, et al: Comparison of the efficacy and safety of valaciclovir and acyclovir for the treatment of herpes zoster ophthalmicus. *Ophthalmology* 2000;107:1507–1511.

Cunningham ET Jr, Margolis TP: Ocular manifestations of HIV infection. *N Engl J Med* 1998; 339:236–244.

Dezube BJ: New therapies for the treatment of AIDS-related Kaposi sarcoma. *Curr Opin Oncol* 2000;12:445–449.

Dugel PU, Gill PS, Frangieh GT, et al: Treatment of ocular adnexal Kaposi's sarcoma in acquired immune deficiency syndrome. *Ophthalmology* 1992;99:1127–1132.

Engstrom RE Jr, Holland GN, Hardy WD, et al: Hemorheologic abnormalities in patients with human immunodeficiency virus infection and ophthalmic microvasculopathy. *Am J Ophthalmol* 1990;109:153–161.

Fogla R, Biswas J, Kumar SK, et al: Squamous cell carcinoma of the conjunctiva as initial presenting sign in a patient with acquired immunodeficiency syndrome (AIDS) due to human immunodeficiency virus type-2. *Eye* 2000;14: 246–247.

Ghabrial R, Quivey JM, Dunn JP Jr, et al: Radiation therapy of acquired immunodeficiency syndrome–related Kaposi's sarcoma of the eyelids and conjunctiva. *Arch Ophthalmol* 1992;110: 1423–1426.

Graham DA, Sires BS: Acquired trichomegaly associated with acquired immunodeficiency syndrome. *Arch Ophthalmol* 1997;115:557–558.

Grossman MC, Cohen PR, Grossman ME: Acquired eyelash trichomegaly and alopecia areata in a human immunodeficiency virus–infected patient. *Dermatology* 1996;193:52–53.

Ingraham HJ, Schoenleber DB: Epibulbar molluscum contagiosum. *Am J Ophthalmol* 1998;125: 394–396.

Jabs DA, Green WR, Fox R, et al: Ocular manifestations of acquired immune deficiency syndrome. *Ophthalmology* 1989;96:1092–1099.

Karbassi M, Raizman MB, Schuman JS: Herpes zoster ophthalmicus. *Surv Ophthalmol* 1992;36: 395–410.

Kestelyn PH, Stevens AM, Ndayambaje A, et al: HIV and conjunctival malignancies. *Lancet* 1990; 336:51–52.

Khan MA, Dhillon B: Epiphora due to Kaposi's sarcoma of the nasolacrimal duct. *Br J Ophthalmol* 1999;83:501–502.

Klutman NE, Hinthorn DR: Excessive growth of eyelashes in a patient with AIDS being treated with zidovudine. *N Engl J Med* 1991;324:1896.

Kronish JW, Johnson TE, Gilberg SM, et al: Orbital infections in patients with human immunodeficiency virus infection. *Ophthalmology* 1996; 103:1483–1492.

Lewallen S, Courtright P: HIV and AIDS and the eye in developing countries: a review. *Arch Ophthalmol* 1997;115:1291–1295.

Lewallen S, Shroyer KR, Keyser RB, et al: Aggressive conjunctival squamous cell carcinoma in three young Africans. *Arch Ophthalmol* 1996;114: 215–218.

Macher AM, Palestine A, Masur H, et al: Multicentric Kaposi's sarcoma of the conjunctiva in a male homosexual with the acquired immunodeficiency syndrome. *Ophthalmology* 1983;90: 879–884.

Mansour AM: Adnexal findings in AIDS. *Ophthalmic Plast Reconstr Surg* 1993;9:273–279.

Margolis TP, Milner MS, Shama A, et al: Herpes zoster ophthalmicus in patients with human immunodeficiency virus infection. *Am J Ophthalmol* 1998;125:285–291.

Meisler DM, Lowder CY, Holland GN: Corneal and external ocular infections in acquired immunodeficiency syndrome (AIDS). In: Krachmer JH, Mannis MJ, Holland EJ, eds: *Cornea. Vol 2: Cornea and External Disease: Clinical Diagnosis and Management.* St Louis: CV Mosby Co; 1997:1017–1022.

Muccioli C, Belfort R Jr: Presumed ocular and central nervous system tuberculosis in a patient with the acquired immunodeficiency syndrome. *Am J Ophthalmol* 1996;121:217–219.

Muccioli C, Belfort R Jr, Neves R, et al: Limbal and choroidal *Cryptococcus* infection in the acquired immunodeficiency syndrome. *Am J Ophthalmol* 1995;120:539–540.

Ryan-Graham MA, Durand M, Pavan-Langston D: AIDS and the anterior segment. *Int Ophthalmol Clin* 1998;38:241–263.

Shuler JD, Engstrom RE Jr, Holland GN: External ocular disease and anterior segment disorders associated with AIDS. *Int Ophthalmol Clin* 1989; 29:98–104.

Shuler JD, Holland GN, Miles SA, et al: Kaposi sarcoma of the conjunctiva and eyelids associated with the acquired immunodeficiency syndrome. *Arch Ophthalmol* 1989;107:858–862.

Tschachler E, Bergstresser PR, Stingl G: HIV-related skin diseases. *Lancet* 1996;348:659–663.

Tufail A, Holland GN, Fisher TC, et al: Increased polymorphonuclear leucocyte rigidity in HIV infected individuals. *Br J Ophthalmol* 2000; 84:727–731.

Tyring S, Engst R, Corriveau C, et al: Famciclovir for ophthalmic zoster: a randomised aciclovir controlled study. *Br J Ophthalmol* 2001;85: 576–581.

Umeh RE: Herpes zoster ophthalmicus and HIV infection in Nigeria. *Int J STD AIDS* 1998; 9:476–479.

Waddell KM, Lewallen S, Lucas SB, et al: Carcinoma of the conjunctiva and HIV infection in Uganda and Malawi. *Br J Ophthalmol* 1996;80: 503–508.

CHAPTER 5

Anterior Segment Manifestations

Anterior segment complications are common in severely immunocompromised HIV-positive individuals, affecting more than half of such patients. Well-recognized complications include keratoconjunctivitis sicca (dry eye), infectious keratitis, corneal drug toxicity, anterior uveitis, and angle-closure glaucoma. The potential for vision loss due to HIV-related anterior segment complications is high, particularly if complications go unrecognized or undertreated. The prevalence of all anterior segment complications of HIV/AIDS decreases dramatically in patients successfully treated with highly active antiretroviral therapy (HAART).

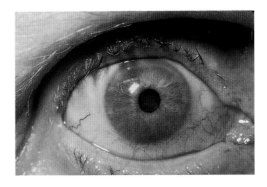

Figure 5-1 *Interpalpebral rose bengal staining in patient with keratoconjunctivitis sicca.*
Courtesy Todd P. Margolis, MD, PhD.

5-1

KERATOCONJUNCTIVITIS SICCA

Keratoconjunctivitis sicca occurs in approximately 10% to 20% of patients infected with HIV, usually during the late stages of the illness. A rapid tear-breakup time, decreased tear meniscus, abnormal Schirmer's test results, and interpalpebral rose bengal staining are typically present (Figure 5-1). The cause of HIV-associated dry eye appears to be multifactorial, but is most probably related to the combined effects of HIV-mediated inflammatory destruction of the primary and accessory lacrimal glands, direct infection and damage of the conjunctiva, and abnormalities in tear composition. Corneal exposure due to lagophthalmos and decreased blink rate in the setting of HIV encephalopathy can worsen corneal changes related to dryness. Patients usually respond to a combination of artificial tears and long-acting lubricating ointments.

5-2

INFECTIOUS KERATITIS

Keratitis may be due to viral, bacterial, fungal, or protozoan infections in patients with HIV disease. As with all corneal infections, prompt diagnosis and treatment optimize the chances for maintenance or recovery of good vision.

5-2-1 Viral Keratitis

5-2-1-1 Varicella Zoster Virus Keratitis Ocular complications occur in more than 50% of HIV-positive patients with herpes zoster ophthalmicus (HZO). As mentioned in Chapter 4, "Adnexal and Orbital Manifestations," HZO refers to a varicella zoster virus (VZV)–related vesiculobullous dermatitis. About one third of HIV-positive patients with HZO develop stromal keratitis, which may present as stromal necrosis, disciform keratitis, stromal edema not in a disciform pattern, avascular stromal infiltrates, or nummular keratitis. A low-grade, self-limiting conjunctivitis, with or without a punctate or dendritic epithelial keratitis, is observed in approximately 15% of patients (Figure 5-2), and a mild-to-moderate ante-

rior uveitis is often present. Up to 5% of patients develop a chronic form of epithelial disease, characterized by severe pain, photophobia, and the presence of multiple slightly raised, pleomorphic pseudodendrites, which may involve the corneal (Figure 5-3), limbal, or bulbar conjunctival epithelium. Both epithelial disease and stromal disease have been described in the absence of skin lesions, a condition termed *herpes zoster sine herpete*. Decreased corneal sensation, acutely elevated intraocular pressure, and iris atrophy and/or transillumination defects provide strong clues to the diagnosis.

Treatment involves acyclovir given either orally (800 mg 5 times daily) or intravenously (10 mg/kg every 8 hours). Intravenous foscarnet may be useful for disease resistant to such therapy. Postherpetic neuralgia may require long-term use of capsaicin or anesthetic cream applied to the skin or an oral tricyclic antidepressant. Maintenance therapy with oral acyclovir (800 mg twice daily) or famciclovir (500 mg 3 times daily) is used to prevent frequent recurrences or when recurrences may irreversibly reduce vision. Maintenance therapy appears to reduce the duration of postherpetic neuralgia.

5-2-1-2 Herpes Simplex Virus Keratitis In contrast to varicella zoster virus (VZV) keratitis, herpes simplex virus (HSV) keratitis seems not to be more common in HIV-positive patients than in the general population. Both epithelial keratitis, which may cause punctate, dendritic (Figure 5-4), or geographic ulcers, and stromal or interstitial disease have been described in HIV-infected individuals. While it has been suggested that HSV epithelial keratitis more commonly in-

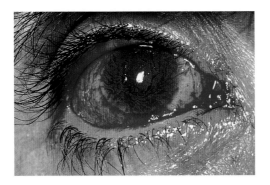

Figure 5-2 *Multiple rose bengal–stained corneal epithelial pseudodendrites in patient with acute VZV keratitis.*
Courtesy Todd P. Margolis, MD, PhD.

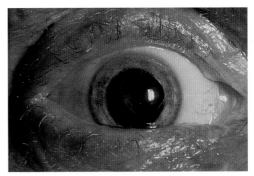

Figure 5-3 *Fluorescein-stained corneal epithelial pseudodendrites in patient with chronic VZV keratitis.*
Reproduced with permission from Cunningham ET Jr, Margolis TP: Ocular manifestations of HIV infection. N Engl J Med *1998;339:236–244. Copyright © 1998 Massachusetts Medical Society. All rights reserved.*

volves the limbus and tends to be characterized by more and larger dendrites in HIV-positive patients, a subsequent study failed to support these findings. However, both studies found that HSV keratitis tends to recur more frequently, and is often more resistant to treatment, in HIV-positive patients as compared to immunocompetent patients.

Both systemic and topical agents may be used to treat HSV keratitis. Systemic treatment options include 7 to 10 days of either oral acyclovir (400 mg 5 times daily) or oral famciclovir (500 mg 3 times daily). Topical treatment options include acyclovir ointment (3% 5 times daily), vidarabine (3% 5 times daily), idoxuridine (0.1% hourly), or trifluridine (1% 9 times daily). Debridement of epithelial lesions may also be performed and can promote healing.

5-2-1-3 Cytomegalovirus Keratitis Although not a true keratitis, asymptomatic corneal endothelial deposits, described clinically as lin-

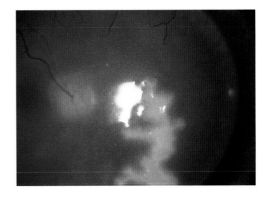

Figure 5-4 *Large limbal dendrite in patient with acute HSV keratitis.*

ear or stellate and often forming a reticular pattern, have been reported in up to 80% of eyes with cytomegalovirus (CMV) retinitis. Best visualized on retroillumination, these findings tend to involve the inferior cornea. Diffuse changes may be observed as well. Histopathologic analysis has revealed these deposits to be composed of fibrin and macrophages, with little evidence of active endothelial infection by CMV.

A single HIV-positive patient with dendritic epithelial keratitis caused by CMV has been described. The patient's disease was resistant to debridement and to both oral and topical antiherpetic therapy. The patient died shortly after diagnosis, with active keratouveitis.

5-2-2 Bacterial and Fungal Keratitis

Both the prevalence of bacterial and fungal keratitis and the composition of ocular flora appear to be similar in HIV-positive and HIV-negative individuals. When bacterial or fungal keratitis does occur, however, it is often more severe, bilateral, associated with multiple pathogens, and has a higher tendency toward perforation in patients with HIV disease. Various bacterial organisms, including *Staphylococcus aureus*, *Staphylococcus epidermidis*, *Pseudomonas aeruginosa*, *Klebsiella oxytoca*, as well as *Streptococcus*, *Bacillus*, *Micrococcus*, and *Capnocytophaga* species, have been identified. *Candida* species have also been reported and appear to be particularly common in HIV-positive drug users. Gram stain, cultures, and sensitivities should be used to guide therapy. Aggressive treatment with hourly topical and subconjunctival fortified antibiotics is indicated in most cases.

5-2-3 Microsporidial Keratitis

Microsporidia are obligate intracellular protozoan parasites known to cause gastroenteritis, hepatitis, peritonitis, sinusitis, pneumonitis, and urogenital infections in patients infected with HIV. Whereas ocular infection in immunocompetent patients is rare and may produce either superficial or deep ulcerative keratitis, only a punctate epithelial keratopathy has been described in HIV-infected patients with ocular microsporidiosis (Figure 5-5), often associated with a mild papillary conjunctivitis. Symptoms are usually mild and may include foreign-body sensation, dryness, photophobia, and blurred vision. The organism is extremely difficult to culture, but can be seen readily within the cytoplasm of corneal or conjunctival epithelial cells using Gram or Giemsa stain (Figure 5-6).

Treatment options include oral itraconazole (200 mg daily), topical propamidine isethionate (Brolene 0.1% 4 times daily), topical fumagillin bicyclohexylammonium salt (70 µg/mL 4 times daily), and oral albendazole (400 to 800 mg daily). Therapy often needs to be continued for 6 to 12 weeks. Microsporidial keratoconjunctivitis has been reported to resolve spontaneously following initiation of HAART.

5-3

CORNEAL DRUG TOXICITY

Ganciclovir, acyclovir, and atovaquone have each been associated with the formation of vortex keratopathy, also termed *corneal phospholipidosis*, in patients with AIDS. Patients are often asymptomatic, but may complain of mild irritation, foreign-body sensation, light sensitivity, or blurred vision. Slit-lamp examination reveals the characteristic whorl-like pattern of gray-white opacities within the corneal epithelium. The appearance may resemble both toxic keratopathy and corneal microsporidiosis, as described above. Vortex keratopathy resolves, albeit slowly, once as the offending agent is discontinued.

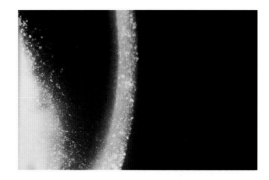

Figure 5-5 *Superficial punctate epithelial keratopathy caused by Microsporidia.*

Reproduced with permission from Cunningham ET Jr, Margolis TP: Ocular manifestations of HIV infection. N Engl J Med 1998;339:236–244. Copyright © 1998 Massachusetts Medical Society. All rights reserved.

5-4

ANTERIOR UVEITIS

Anterior uveitis is common in patients infected with HIV, affecting more than 50% of patients at some time during the course of their illness. While HIV infection alone may cause anterior chamber inflammation, mild iridocyclitis is most often secondary to viral retinitis caused by CMV, VZV, or HSV. More severe anterior chamber inflammation can occur in association with toxoplasmic retinochoroiditis, syphilitic chorioretinitis, and bacterial or fungal retinitis or endophthalmitis. Patients with isolated iridocyclitis caused by toxoplasmosis, cryptococcosis, or syphilis have been described as well. Treatment should be directed toward the specific infectious agent.

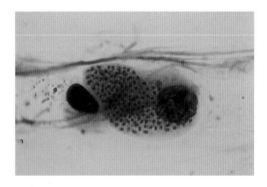

Figure 5-6 *Giemsa stain of two adjacent conjunctival epithelial cells, revealing numerous intracellular Microsporidia.*

Courtesy Vickie Cevallos.

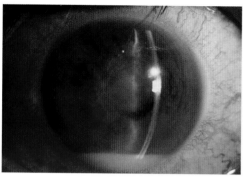

Figure 5-7 *Severe anterior uveitis with fibrin exudate and hypopyon and posterior synechiae formation in patient taking rifabutin.*
Courtesy Janet L. Davis, MD.

Medications may also cause uveitis in HIV-positive patients. For example, rifabutin, which is used to treat *Mycobacterium avium* complex, produces iridocyclitis in up to one third of patients, particularly when used at 600 mg daily or in combination with clarithromycin or fluconazole. Rifabutin-associated hypopyon formation is particularly common (Figure 5-7). Cidofovir, which is given for CMV retinitis, causes severe anterior chamber inflammation in nearly 50% of patients. Lastly, terbinafine, which is used to treat oral candidiasis, has been associated with uveitis in isolated patients.

Treatment includes reducing the dose or discontinuing the offending agent while controlling active inflammation, minimizing discomfort, and reducing the risk of posterior synechiae formation with a topical corticosteroid, such as prednisolone acetate 1%, and a cycloplegic/mydriatic agent, such as Cyclogyl 1% or homatropine 5%.

HAART is associated with uveitis, which may involve the anterior chamber in up to two thirds of patients with a history of CMV retinitis who experience immune recovery. Vitreous inflammation is the most salient clinical feature, however (see Chapter 6, "Posterior Segment Manifestations").

5-5

ANGLE-CLOSURE GLAUCOMA

Acute angle-closure glaucoma has been described in association with uveal effusion syndrome in patients infected with HIV. Peripheral iridotomies have little effect, and, paradoxically, miotics worsen the condition. Intraocular inflammation is minimal or absent, but, if pronounced, should raise suspicion of primary choroidal inflammation with secondary exudative retinal detachments. Choroidal effusions are usually visible clinically, although ultrasonography may be required to demonstrate shallow anterior detachments. The cause of HIV-associated angle-closure glaucoma is unknown. Axial length should be checked in all patients to exclude the possibility of nanophthalmos.

Treatment includes cycloplegics, corticosteroids, aqueous suppressants, hyperosmolar agents, and, when necessary, surgical drainage of suprachoroidal fluid.

SELECTED REFERENCES

Acharya NR, Cunningham ET Jr: Corneal, anterior segment, and adnexal manifestations of human immunodeficiency virus. *Int Ophthalmol Clin* 1998;38:161–177.

Akduman L, Pepose JS: Anterior segment manifestations of acquired immunodeficiency syndrome. *Sem Ophthalmol* 1995;10:111–118.

Akler ME, Johnson DW, Burman WJ, et al: Anterior uveitis and hypotony after intravenous cidofovir for the treatment of cytomegalovirus retinitis. *Ophthalmology* 1998;105:651–657.

Ambati J, Wynne KB, Angerame MC, et al: Anterior uveitis associated with intravenous cidofovir use in patients with cytomegalovirus retinitis. *Br J Ophthalmol* 1999;83:1153–1158.

Brody JM, Butrus SI, Laby DM, et al: Anterior segment findings in AIDS patients with cytomegalovirus retinitis. *Graefes Arch Clin Exp Ophthalmol* 1995;233:374–376.

Cano-Parra JL, Diaz-LLopis ML, Cordoba JL, et al: Acute iridocyclitis in a patient with AIDS diagnosed as toxoplasmosis by PCR [polymerase chain reaction]. *Ocul Immunol Inflamm* 2000;8:127–130.

Chavez–de la Paz E, Arevalo JF, Kirsch LS, et al: Anterior nongranulomatous uveitis after intravitreal HPMPC (cidofovir) for the treatment of cytomegalovirus retinitis: analysis and prevention. *Ophthalmology* 1997;104:539–544.

Chern KC, Conrad D, Holland GN, et al: Chronic varicella-zoster virus epithelial keratitis in patients with acquired immunodeficiency syndrome. *Arch Ophthalmol* 1998;116:1011–1017.

Chern KC, Margolis TP: Varicella zoster virus ocular disease. *Int Ophthalmol Clin* 1998;38:149–160.

Cochereau I, Doan S, Diraison MC, et al: Uveitis in patients treated with intravenous cidofovir. *Ocul Immunol Inflamm* 1999;7:223–229.

Cole EL, Meisler DM, Calabrese LH, et al: Herpes zoster ophthalmicus and acquired immune deficiency syndrome. *Arch Ophthalmol* 1984;102:1027–1029.

Couderc LJ, D'Agay MF, Danon F, et al: Sicca complex and infection with human immunodeficiency virus. *Arch Intern Med* 1987;147:898–901.

Cunningham ET Jr: Uveitis in HIV positive patients. *Br J Ophthalmol* 2000;84:233–235.

Cunningham ET Jr, Margolis TP: Ocular manifestations of HIV infection. *N Engl J Med* 1998;339:236–244.

Davis JL, Taskintuna I, Freeman WR, et al: Iritis and hypotony after treatment with intravenous cidofovir for cytomegalovirus retinitis. *Arch Ophthalmol* 1997;115:733–737.

Fineman MS, Emerick G, Dudley D, et al: Bilateral choroidal effusions and angle-closure glaucoma associated with human immunodeficiency virus infection. *Retina* 1997;17:455–457.

Font RL, Samaha AN, Keener MJ, et al: Corneal microsporidiosis: report of case, including electron microscopic observations. *Ophthalmology* 2000;107:1769–1775.

Gordon JJ, Golbus J, Kurtides ES: Chronic lymphadenopathy and Sjogren's syndrome in a homosexual man. *N Engl J Med* 1984;311: 1441–1442.

Gritz DC, Scott TJ, Sedo SF, et al: Ocular flora of patients with AIDS compared with those of HIV-negative patients. *Cornea* 1997;16:400–405.

Hemady RK: Microbial keratitis in patients infected with the human immunodeficiency virus. *Ophthalmology* 1995;102:1026–1030.

Henderson HW, Mitchell SM: Treatment of immune recovery vitritis with local steroids. *Br J Ophthalmol* 1999;83:540–545.

Hodge WG, Margolis TP: Herpes simplex virus keratitis among patients who are positive or negative for human immunodeficiency virus: an epidemiologic study. *Ophthalmology* 1997;104: 120–124.

Holland GN: Immune recovery uveitis. *Ocul Immunol Inflamm* 1999;7:215–221.

Itescu S, Brancato LJ, Buxbaum J, et al: A diffuse infiltrative CD8 lymphocytosis syndrome in human immunodeficiency virus (HIV) infection: a host immune response associated with HLA-DR5. *Ann Intern Med* 1990;112:3–10.

Karavellas MP, Azen SP, MacDonald JC, et al: Immune recovery vitritis and uveitis in AIDS: clinical predictors, sequelae, and treatment outcomes. *Retina* 2001;21:1–9.

Karavellas MP, Song M, Macdonald JC, et al: Long-term posterior and anterior segment complications of immune recovery uveitis associated with cytomegalovirus retinitis. *Am J Ophthalmol* 2000;130:57–64.

Krzystolik MG, Kuperwasser M, Low RM, et al: Anterior-segment ultrasound biomicroscopy in a patient with AIDS and bilateral angle-closure glaucoma secondary to uveal effusions. *Arch Ophthalmol* 1996;114:878–879.

Kuppermann BD, Holland GN: Immune recovery uveitis. *Am J Ophthalmol* 2000;130:103–106.

Lee-Wing MW, Hodge WG, Diaz-Mitoma F: Investigating a viral etiology for keratoconjunctivitis sicca among patients who are positive for human immunodeficiency virus. *Cornea* 1999;18: 671–674.

Lowder CY, McMahon JT, Meisler DM, et al: Microsporidial keratoconjunctivitis caused by *Septata intestinalis* in a patient with acquired immunodeficiency syndrome. *Am J Ophthalmol* 1996;121:715–717.

Lucca JA, Farris RL, Bielory L, et al: Keratoconjunctivitis sicca in male patients infected with human immunodeficiency virus type 1. *Ophthalmology* 1990;97:1008–1010.

Lucca JA, Kung JS, Farris RL: Keratoconjunctivitis sicca in female patients infected with human immunodeficiency virus. *CLAO J* 1994; 20:49–51.

Lucca JA, Kung JS, Farris RL: Keratoconjunctivitis sicca in HIV-1 infected female patients. *Adv Exp Med Biol* 1994;350:521–523.

Margolis TP, Milner MS, Shama A, et al: Herpes zoster ophthalmicus in patients with human immunodeficiency virus infection. *Am J Ophthalmol* 1998;125:285–291.

Martins SA, Muccioli C, Belfort R Jr, et al: Resolution of microsporidial keratoconjunctivitis in an AIDS patient treated with highly active antiretroviral therapy. *Am J Ophthalmol* 2001;131: 378–379.

Meillet D, Hoang PL, Unanue F, et al: Filtration and local synthesis of lacrimal proteins in acquired immunodeficiency syndrome. *Eur J Clin Chem Clin Biochem* 1992;30:319–323.

Meisler DM, Lowder CY, Holland GN: Corneal and external ocular infections in acquired immunodeficiency syndrome (AIDS). In: Krachmer JH, Mannis MJ, Holland EJ, eds: *Cornea. Vol 2: Cornea and External Disease: Clinical Diagnosis and Management.* St Louis: CV Mosby Co; 1997:1017–1022.

Mselle J: Fungal keratitis as an indicator of HIV infection in Africa. *Trop Doctor* 1999;29:133–135.

Nguyen QD, Kempen JH, Bolton SG, et al: Immune recovery uveitis in patients with AIDS and cytomegalovirus retinitis after highly active antiretroviral therapy. *Am J Ophthalmol* 2000;129:634–639.

Nussenblatt RB, Lane HC: Human immunodeficiency virus disease: changing patterns of intraocular inflammation. *Am J Ophthalmol* 1998;125:374–382.

Pepose JS: The potential impact of the varicella vaccine and new antivirals on ocular disease related to varicella-zoster virus. *Am J Ophthalmol* 1997;123:243–251.

Pflugfelder SC, Saulson R, Ullman S: Peripheral corneal ulceration in a patient with AIDS-related complex. *Am J Ophthalmol* 1987;104:542–543.

Pimentel L, Booth D, Greenwood J, et al: Secondary acute angle closure glaucoma: a complication of AIDS. *J Emerg Med* 1997;15:811–814.

Price T, Stallman J, Dretler RH: Anterior uveitis in a patient with AIDS who was treated with terbinafine for oral candidiasis: a potential drug-induced reaction. *Clin Infect Dis* 1997;25:752–753.

Robinson MR, Reed G, Csaky KG, et al: Immune-recovery uveitis in patients with cytomegalovirus retinitis taking highly active antiretroviral therapy. *Am J Ophthalmol* 2000;130:49–56.

Robinson MR, Ross ML, Whitcup SM: Ocular manifestations of HIV infection. *Curr Opin Ophthalmol* 1999;10:431–437.

Rosberger DF, Heinemann MH, Friedberg DN, et al: Uveitis associated with human immunodeficiency virus infection. *Am J Ophthalmol* 1998;125:301–305.

Ryan-Graham MA, Durand M, Pavan-Langston D: AIDS and the anterior segment. *Int Ophthalmol Clin* 1998;38:241–263.

Sandor EV, Millman A, Croxson TS, et al: Herpes zoster ophthalmicus in patients at risk for the acquired immune deficiency syndrome (AIDS). *Am J Ophthalmol* 1986;101:153–155.

Shah GK, Cantrill HL, Holland EJ: Vortex keratopathy associated with atovaquone. *Am J Ophthalmol* 1995;120:669–671.

Shuler JD, Engstrom RE Jr, Holland GN: External ocular disease and anterior segment disorders associated with AIDS. *Int Ophthalmol Clin* 1989;29:98–104.

Tseng AL, Walmsley SL: Rifabutin-associated uveitis. *Ann Pharmacother* 1995;29:1149–1155.

Ulirsch RC, Jaffe ES: Sjogren's syndrome–like illness associated with the acquired immunodeficiency syndrome–related complex. *Hum Pathol* 1987;18:1063–1068.

Vrabec TR: Advances in the diagnosis and management of AIDS-related eye disease. *Curr Opin Ophthalmol* 1998;9:93–99.

Walter KA, Coulter VL, Palay DA, et al: Corneal endothelial deposits in patients with cytomegalovirus retinitis. *Am J Ophthalmol* 1996;121:391–396.

Wilhelmus KR, Font RL, Lehmann RP, et al: Cytomegalovirus keratitis in acquired immunodeficiency syndrome. *Arch Ophthalmol* 1996;114:869–872.

Wilhelmus KR, Keener MJ, Jones DB, et al: Corneal lipidosis in patients with the acquired immunodeficiency syndrome. *Am J Ophthalmol* 1995;119:14–19.

Young TL, Robin JB, Holland GN, et al: Herpes simplex keratitis in patients with acquired immune deficiency syndrome. *Ophthalmology* 1989;96:1476–1479.

Zambarakji HJ, Simcock PR: Bilateral angle closure glaucoma in HIV infection. *J Roy Soc Med* 1996;89:581–582.

Zegans ME, Walton RC, Holland GN, et al: Transient vitreous inflammatory reactions associated with combination antiretroviral therapy in patients with AIDS and cytomegalovirus retinitis. *Am J Ophthalmol* 1998;125:292–300.

Posterior Segment Manifestations

Posterior segment complications of HIV infection are common and often visually important. Retinal microvasculopathy and cytomegalovirus (CMV) retinitis together account for the majority of the ocular complications in HIV-positive individuals. Moreover, CMV retinitis is the single most significant cause of loss of vision in this population, affecting up to 40% of untreated HIV-positive patients. As with adnexal and anterior segment complications, the prevalence of all posterior segment complications of HIV/AIDS decreases dramatically in patients successfully treated with highly active antiretroviral therapy (HAART).

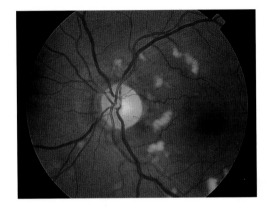

Figure 6-1 *HIV retinopathy with numerous cotton-wool spots.*

RETINAL MICROVASCULOPATHY

Prior to HAART, retinal microvasculopathy occurred in up to 50% of untreated HIV-infected patients. The most commonly observed manifestation is cotton-wool spots (Figure 6-1), although intraretinal hemorrhages, microaneurysms, and retinal ischemia may also occur. With the exception of retinal ischemia, these findings are transient and rarely affect vision. All forms of retinal microvasculopathy increase in frequency in the more advanced stages of HIV infection. Hypotheses regarding the pathogenesis of retinal microvasculopathy parallel those suggested for conjunctival vascular changes: HIV-induced increase in plasma viscosity, HIV-related immune complex deposition, and direct infection of the conjunctival vascular endothelium by HIV.

Retinal microvasculopathy associated with HIV is typically asymptomatic, but may contribute to the progressive optic nerve atrophy, electroretinographic abnormalities, loss of color vision, decreased contrast sensitivity, and visual field changes observed in HIV-infected patients. The role of retinal microvasculopathy in the development of CMV retinitis is controversial, with some investigators finding no relationship and others suggesting that retinal vascular damage may provide increased access to circulating CMV-infected lymphocytes.

6-2

INFECTIOUS RETINITIS

6-2-1 Cytomegalovirus Retinitis

CMV retinitis affects up to 40% of untreated HIV-positive patients, typically as CD4$^+$ T-lymphocyte counts fall below 100 cells/μL. Any portion of the fundus may be involved, including the optic nerve head, which is affected in approximately 5% to 10% of cases. Patients with CMV retinitis typically describe gradual visual field loss or the onset of floaters. Clinical examination shows geographic thickening and opacification of the retina. Three clinical presentations have been described:

1. Granular CMV retinitis, which tends to be less edematous and has few intraretinal hemorrhages (Figure 6-2)

2. Fulminant or hemorrhagic CMV retinitis, which is more edematous and often has numerous and/or extensive intraretinal hemorrhages (Figure 6-3)

3. Perivascular CMV retinitis, which resembles frosted-branch angiitis originally described in immunocompetent children (Figure 6-4)

While the natural history and prognosis appear to be similar for these various presentations of CMV retinitis, recognizing the particular form is important for prompt diagnosis and treatment. Anterior chamber and vitreous inflammation, although invariably observed, is usually mild. Retinal detachment occurs in roughly one third of patients and often requires vitrectomy and silicone-oil placement to achieve lasting repair.

Treatment of CMV retinitis is complicated and needs to be tailored to each pa-

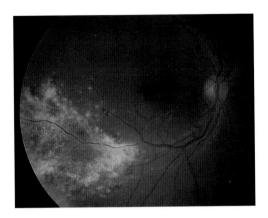

Figure 6-2 *Granular CMV retinitis. Note multiple satellite lesions at advancing edge.*

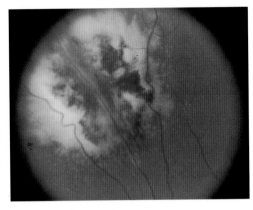

Figure 6-3 *Fulminant or hemorrhagic CMV retinitis. Retinal edema and hemorrhages are more pronounced.*

tient (Table 6-1). Currently available FDA-approved treatment options for active retinitis include intravenous ganciclovir, intravenous foscarnet, intravenous cidofovir, and valganciclovir, the oral pro-drug of ganciclovir. Intravitreous fomivirsen, a 21-nucleotide phosphorthioate oligonucleotide that works by an antisense mechanism, is FDA-approved to treat reactivations and is reserved most often for CMV retinitis that has been resistant to other therapies. Any of these drugs or the oral formulation of ganciclovir can be used for maintenance therapy. Local therapy with intravitreal injection of ganciclovir or foscarnet or via implantation of a slow-release ganciclovir-containing reservoir is also possible. The choice of an appropriate antiviral drug and route of delivery needs to be individualized and should be based on consideration of the location and extent of ocular and systemic disease, an understanding of potential drug-related side effects, and knowledge of viral response to past treatments.

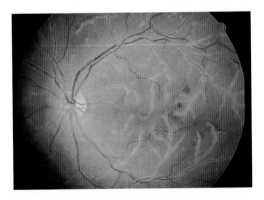

Figure 6-4 *Perivascular CMV retinitis, mimicking frosted-branch retinitis.*
Courtesy J. Michael Lahey, MD.

TABLE 6-1

Treatment Options for Cytomegalovirus Retinitis

Drug*	Dosage*	Systemic Monitoring	Side Effects
Intravenous ganciclovir	Induction: 5–7.5 mg/kg every 12 hr for 2–3 wk Maintenance: 5 mg/kg daily	Complete blood cell count twice weekly during induction, weekly thereafter Serum creatinine monthly	Neutropenia (10%–15%) Thrombocytopenia (5%) Catheter infection (<1%)
Oral ganciclovir	1 g 3 times daily	Complete blood cell count weekly Serum creatinine monthly	Neutropenia (<10%) Thrombocytopenia (<10%)
Intravitreous ganciclovir injection	400–2000 µg in 0.1-cc volume twice weekly until inactive, weekly thereafter	NA	Retinal detachment (<5%) Vitreous hemorrhage (<5%) Endophthalmitis (<1%)
Intravitreous ganciclovir implant	4.5 g	NA	Same as ganciclovir injection
Intravenous foscarnet	Induction: 90 mg/kg every 12 hr for 2–3 wk Maintenance: 90 mg/kg daily	Serum creatinine, potassium, magnesium, calcium, phosphorous twice weekly during induction, weekly thereafter	Transient hypocalcemia during infusion Nephrotoxicity (10%–20%)
Intravitreous foscarnet injection	2400 µg in 0.1-cc volume twice weekly until inactive, weekly thereafter	NA	Same as ganciclovir injection

*May be contraindicated or dose may need to be reduced for patients prone to dehydration, with reduced creatinine clearance, with documented neutropenia or thrombocytopenia, or concurrently taking other myelotoxic or nephrotoxic drugs.

Source: *Modified with permission from Cunningham ET Jr, Margolis TP: Ocular manifestations of HIV infection.* N Engl J Med *1998;339:236–244. Copyright © 1998 Massachusetts Medical Society. All rights reserved.*

Median Time to Progression	Advantages	Disadvantages	Relative Indications
1.5–2.5 months	Provides treatment and protection for fellow eye and distant organs	Systemic side effects common Requires daily infusions	Bilateral or systemic treatment required Non–vision-threatening lesions, not involving zone 1[†]
1.5 months	Provides treatment and protection for fellow eye and distant organs	Frequent daily dosing Lower systemic and intraocular drug levels and shorter median time to progression compared to intravenous therapy	Protection for fellow eye or distant organs in setting of local injection or implant therapy Maintenance therapy for non–vision-threatening lesions
NA	Immediate, high-dose intraocular drug delivery	Frequent injections No treatment or protection for fellow eye or distant organs	Vision-threatening lesions (zone 1) Systemic medications contraindicated, poorly tolerated, or show poor response[‡]
6–8 months (duration of drug)	High-dose intraocular drug delivery Long duration	No treatment or protection for fellow eye or distant organs Moderate, transient visual loss for 4–6 wk after surgery	Same as injection
1–2 months	Same as intravenous ganciclovir	Same as intravenous ganciclovir	Same as intravenous ganciclovir When systemic ganciclovir is contraindicated or shows poor response
NA	Same as ganciclovir injection	Same as ganciclovir injection	Same as ganciclovir injection When systemic or intravitreous therapy shows poor response

[†]*Zone 1 is defined as within 1500 μm of optic nerve head or 3000 μm of fovea.*

[‡]*Response to therapy may be poor due to low intraocular drug levels, poor penetration or compliance, relative viral resistance, or misdiagnosis. Toxoplasmosis, other herpes virus infections (such as varicella zoster virus and herpes simplex virus), bacterial infections (such as syphilis), fungal infections (such as* Candida*), and intraocular lymphoma should be considered in every HIV-positive patient with retinitis who shows poor initial response to anti-CMV therapy.*

(continued)

TABLE 6-1 *(cont.)*

Treatment Options for Cytomegalovirus Retinitis

Drug*	Dosage*	Systemic Monitoring	Side Effects
Combined intravenous ganciclovir and foscarnet	Induction: *either* 90 mg/kg foscarnet twice daily plus 5 mg/kg ganciclovir once daily *or* 5 mg/kg ganciclovir twice daily plus 90 mg/kg foscarnet once daily for 2–3 wk Maintenance: 90 mg/kg foscarnet with 5 mg/kg ganciclovir daily	Same as each drug alone	Same as each drug alone
Intravenous cidofovir	Induction: 5 mg/kg weekly for 2–3 wk Maintenance: 5 mg/kg every 2 wk Probenecid 2 g 3 hr before infusion and 1 g 2 and 8 hr after infusion	Serum creatinine, urinary protein, and complete blood cell count before each infusion	Nephrotoxicity (25%) Uveitis (25%–30%) Low intraocular pressure (10%) Neutropenia Peripheral neuropathy
Oral valganciclovir	Induction: 450 mg twice daily for 21 days Maintenance: 450 mg once daily	Same as intravenous ganciclovir	Same as intravenous ganciclovir
Intravitreous fomivirsen	Induction: 165 µg/0.1 mL to 330 µg/0.1 mL weekly for 3 wk Maintenance: 165 µg/0.1 mL to 330 µg/0.1 mL every other week	NA	Same as ganciclovir or foscarnet injection Elevated intraocular pressure, moderate uveitis, bull's-eye maculopathy

Median Time to Progression	Advantages	Disadvantages	Relative Indications
4–5 months	Longer time to progression Maximal treatment and protection for fellow eye and distant organs	Combined side effects Long daily infusion times	Severe or systemic infection poorly responsive to either drug alone
3 months	Decreased total infusion time Eliminates need for indwelling catheter Provides treatment and protection for fellow eye and distant organs Increased median time to progression compared to other systemic agents	Potential for severe nephrotoxicity, especially in patients with prior kidney disease or who are prone to dehydration Uveitis and low intraocular pressure may limit therapy in significant percentage of patients	Daily infusions contraindicated or poorly tolerated When systemic ganciclovir and foscarnet are contraindicated, poorly tolerated, or show poor response
Same as intravenous ganciclovir	Same as intravenous ganciclovir	Same as intravenous ganciclovir, but avoids daily infusion	Same as intravenous ganciclovir Patient unable to tolerate daily intravenous therapy
2–3 months	Same as injection Most useful in otherwise unresponsive forms of CMV retinitis	Same as injection Unique inflammatory, intraocular pressure, and retinal pigmentary complications	CMV retinitis unresponsive to other forms of therapy

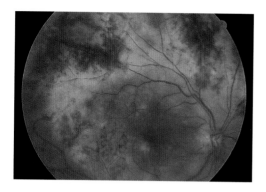

Figure 6-5 *VZV retinitis causing PORN.*

Withdrawing CMV therapy may be considered for patients who experience immune reconstitution while being treated with HAART once viral loads are low and stable and CD4$^+$ T-lymphocyte counts exceed 100 cells/μL on at least two separate testings over a 3-month period. Discontinuing CMV retinitis therapy should be done with caution, however, particularly in patients with bilateral disease, with CMV retinitis near or involving the optic disc or macula (zone 1), or with loss of vision in one eye. Because drug intolerance and viral resistance are common with HAART, patients need to be monitored at regular intervals, even after CD4$^+$ T-lymphocyte counts rise.

6-2-2 Varicella Zoster Virus Retinitis

Varicella zoster virus (VZV) is the second most common cause of necrotizing retinitis in HIV-infected individuals, affecting approximately 5% of large untreated cohorts with AIDS. Like CMV, VZV produces retinal whitening, occasionally accompanied by intraretinal hemorrhages. VZV retinitis is usually distinguished by its rapid progression and the simultaneous occurrence of multiple large confluent areas of retinitis (Figure 6-5). The VZV retinitis that occurs in profoundly immunosuppressed patients is often termed *progressive outer retinal necrosis* (PORN) and tends to have much less vitreous inflammation than the VZV retinitis that occurs in partly immunocompromised or immunocompetent patients, also known as *acute retinal necrosis* (ARN). Concurrent or recent herpes zoster dermatitis provides added circumstantial support for

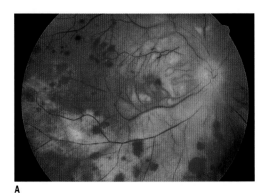

A

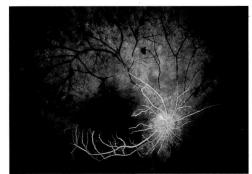

B

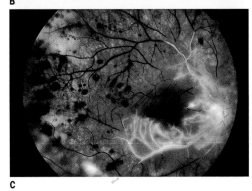

C

the diagnosis. Concurrent or subsequent involvement of the fellow eye is common. Retinal detachment occurs in up to two thirds of involved eyes.

Many authorities recommend treatment with combined intravenous acyclovir (10 mg/kg every 8 hours) and twice weekly intravitreous foscarnet (2.4 mg/0.1 mL) or ganciclovir (2.0 mg/0.1 mL) until the retinitis shows obvious improvement. Most patients are then maintained on oral antiviral therapy, as described in Chapter 4, "Adnexal and Orbital Manifestations," for herpes zoster ophthalmicus, at least as long as their CD4+ T-lymphocyte counts remain low. The visual prognosis remains guarded, however, even with prompt and aggressive treatment.

6-2-3 Herpes Simplex Virus Retinitis

Herpes simplex virus (HSV) is a rare cause of retinitis in patients infected with HIV. The clinical appearance of HSV retinitis may mimic VZV retinitis in all respects, however, including rapid progression and profound loss of vision (Figure 6-6). While

Figure 6-6 *HSV type 1 retinitis (A) causing PORN. (B) Early and (C) late fluorescein angiograms reveal extensive vascular occlusion of actively inflamed retinal vessels.*

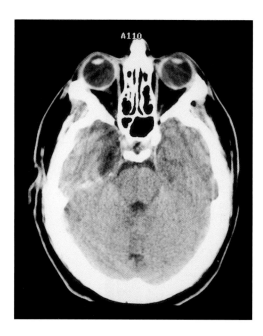

Figure 6-7 *Magnetic resonance imaging (MRI) scan of HSV encephalitis involving right temporal lobe in patient with HSV retinitis.*

the occurrence of prior or concurrent encephalitis can help distinguish HSV retinitis from VZV retinitis (Figure 6-7), definitive diagnosis usually involves polymerase chain reaction–based amplification of HSV-specific DNA from vitreous biopsy fluid.

As with VZV retinitis, treatment of HSV retinitis should include combined intravenous acyclovir and intravitreous foscarnet or ganciclovir, followed by oral maintenance therapy.

6-2-4 Toxoplasmic Retinochoroiditis

Ocular toxoplasmosis affects less than 1% of patients infected with HIV in the United States, but is more common in regions with a high seroprevalence of anti-*Toxoplasma* serum antibodies, such as Brazil and France. Toxoplasmic retinochoroiditis in HIV-positive patients is usually distinguished by a moderate-to-severe anterior chamber and vitreous inflammation (Figure 6-8), a relative lack of retinal hemorrhage, and a smooth rather than granular leading edge. Moreover, HIV-infected individuals may have multifocal or bilateral disease, with no evidence of inactive retinochoroidal scars—a presentation that appears to be less common in immunocompetent patients. Testing should include serology for immunoglobin G (IgG) and immunoglobin M (IgM) anti-*Toxoplasma* antibodies, but the test results may be negative in profoundly immunosuppressed patients. A sizable proportion of HIV-positive patients with toxoplasmic retinochoroiditis have central nervous system involvement, which is best evaluated with contrast-enhanced magnetic resonance imaging (MRI).

Treatment of active retinitis consists of a sulfonamide and pyrimethamine, often in

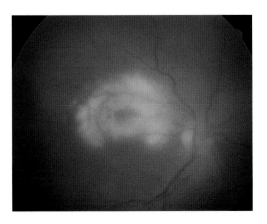

Figure 6-8 *Toxoplasmic retinochoroiditis with moderately severe vitreous inflammation.*

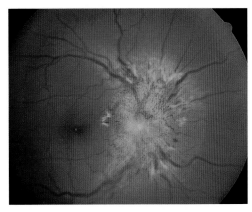

Figure 6-9 *Papillitis due to syphilis.*

combination with clindamycin. Azathioprine has also been used, but has been associated with treatment failures. Long-term or intermittent therapy is often necessary, but can be complicated by side effects. Sulfa allergies, in particular, are quite common in patients with HIV/AIDS. Atovaquone has been used with success to treat toxoplasmic retinochoroiditis in HIV-positive patients, but is expensive and has yet to be shown to be superior to more standard combination therapy.

6-2-5 Bacterial and Fungal Retinitis

Ocular syphilis is the most common intraocular bacterial infection, affecting up to 2% of HIV-positive individuals. Patients may present with either an iridocyclitis or a more diffuse intraocular inflammation, with or without retinal or optic nerve involvement (Figure 6-9). Laboratory testing should include both a rapid plasma reagin (RPR) test or a Venereal Disease Research Laboratory (VDRL) test and a specific treponemal antibody test: fluorescent treponemal antibody absorption (FTA-ABS) test or microhemagglutination assay for *Treponema pallidum* (MHA-TP). However, these tests may be negative in HIV-positive individuals, despite active intraocular disease. Treatment includes intravenous penicillin G, 24 million units/day for 7 to 14 days. Recurrences can occur despite adequate treatment in individuals infected with HIV.

Other bacterial and fungal causes of retinitis or endophthalmitis are rare in patients infected with HIV, but have included *Staphylococcus aureus* and *Histoplasma capsulatum* among other species. Neuroretinitis associated with systemic *Bartonella henselae* infection has also been described in patients with HIV disease.

6-3

INFECTIOUS CHOROIDITIS

Infectious choroiditis is uncommon in HIV-infected patients, accounting for less than 1% of all ocular findings in most clinic-based series. Clinically, the most common causes are *Pneumocystis carinii* (Figure 6-10), *Cryptococcus neoformans* (Figure 6-11), and

Mycobacterium tuberculosis (Figure 6-12). *Mycobacterium avium* complex, *Histoplasma capsulatum*, *Candida*, and *Aspergillus fumigatus* have also been reported in autopsy series. Up to one third of HIV-positive patients with choroiditis also have evidence of active or inactive CMV retinitis.

6-4

INTRAOCULAR LYMPHOMA

Although uncommon, HIV-infected patients are at increased risk for developing primary intraocular lymphoma. Lesions are usually subretinal, numerous, and tend to be yellow-white. A mild-to-moderate vitritis is often present. HIV-associated intraocular lymphomas are usually composed primarily of B cells, although T-cell tumors have also been described. Treatment includes combination radiation and chemotherapy.

6-5

RETINAL VEIN OR ARTERY OCCLUSION

Large retinal vessel occlusion occurs in less than 1% of patients with AIDS and appears to be more common in severely immunosuppressed individuals. Retinal veins (Figure 6-13) appear to be affected more often than retinal arteries. The cause is unknown, but may be related to the same rheologic and vascular factors that contribute to HIV retinopathy.

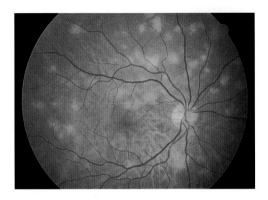

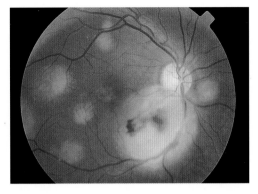

Figure 6-10 Pneumocystis carinii *choroiditis. Similar findings were present in fellow eye.*

Figure 6-11 Cryptococcus neoformans *choroiditis. Similar findings were present in fellow eye. Courtesy J. Michael Lahey, MD.*

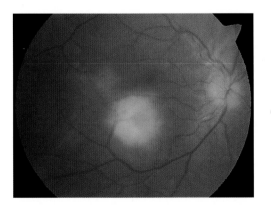

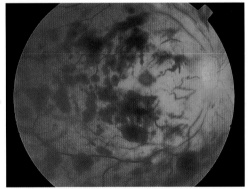

Figure 6-12 Mycobacterium tuberculosis *choroiditis. Courtesy Cristina Muccioli, MD.*

Figure 6-13 *Central retinal vein occlusion.*

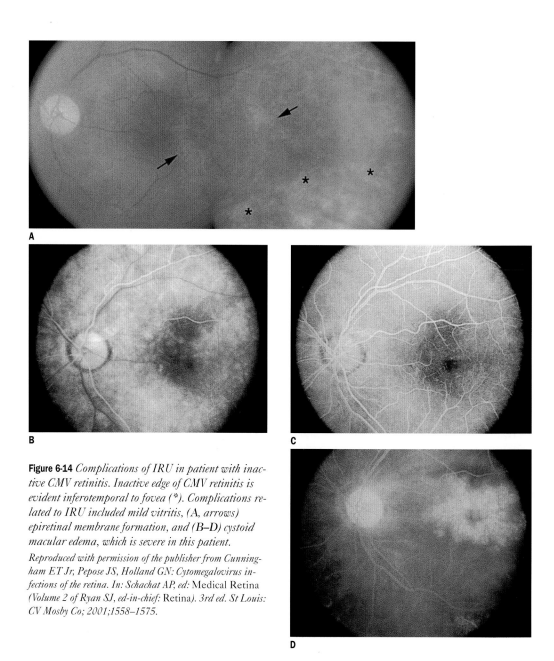

Figure 6-14 *Complications of IRU in patient with inactive CMV retinitis. Inactive edge of CMV retinitis is evident inferotemporal to fovea (*). Complications related to IRU included mild vitritis, (A, arrows) epiretinal membrane formation, and (B–D) cystoid macular edema, which is severe in this patient.*

Reproduced with permission of the publisher from Cunningham ET Jr, Pepose JS, Holland GN: Cytomegalovirus infections of the retina. In: Schachat AP, ed: Medical Retina *(Volume 2 of Ryan SJ, ed-in-chief:* Retina*). 3rd ed. St Louis: CV Mosby Co; 2001;1558–1575.*

6-6

IMMUNE RECOVERY UVEITIS

Immune recovery uveitis (IRU) has been recognized only since the advent of HAART. This paradoxical worsening of intraocular inflammation is observed in eyes with clinically inactive CMV retinitis and appears to occur more often in eyes that have had extensive retinal involvement. Secondary vision-threatening complications that can occur in patients with IRU include moderate-to-severe vitreous inflammation, traction retinal detachment, retinal neovascularization, epiretinal membrane formation, and cystoid macular edema (Figure 6-14).

Treatment typically involves combined use of topical and periocular corticosteroids, which may need to be prolonged or repeated. Surgery may be required for patients with vision loss caused by epiretinal membrane formation or traction retinal detachment.

SELECTED REFERENCES

Akduman L, Feiner MA, Olk RJ, et al: Macular ischemia as a cause of decreased vision in a patient with acquired immunodeficiency syndrome. *Am J Ophthalmol* 1997;124:699–702.

Antle CM, White VA, Horsman DE, et al: Large cell orbital lymphoma in a patient with acquired immune deficiency syndrome: case report and review. *Ophthalmology* 1990;97:1494–1498.

Bogie GJ, Nanda SK: Neovascularization associated with cytomegalovirus retinitis. *Retina* 2001; 21:85–87.

Brooks HL Jr, Downing J, McClure JA, et al: Orbital Burkitt's lymphoma in a homosexual man with acquired immune deficiency. *Arch Ophthalmol* 1984;102:1533–1537.

Canzano JC, Reed JB, Morse LS: Vitreomacular traction syndrome following highly active antiretroviral therapy in AIDS patients with cytomegalovirus retinitis. *Retina* 1998;18:443–447.

Cassoux N, Bodaghi B, Fillet AM, et al: Relapses of CMV retinitis after 2 years of highly active antiretroviral therapy. *Br J Ophthalmol* 2000;84:1203.

Cassoux N, Bodaghi B, Katlama C, et al: CMV retinitis in the era of HAART. *Ocul Immunol Inflamm* 1999;7:231–235.

Conway MD, Tong P, Olk RJ: Branch retinal artery occlusion (BRAO) combined with branch retinal vein occlusion (BRVO) and optic disc neovascularization associated with HIV and CMV retinitis. *Int Ophthalmol* 1995–96;19: 249–252.

Cunningham ET Jr: Uveitis in HIV positive patients. *Br J Ophthalmol* 2000;84:233–235.

Cunningham ET Jr, Margolis TP: Ocular manifestations of HIV infection. *N Engl J Med* 1998; 339:236–244.

Cunningham ET Jr, Pepose JS, Holland GN: Cytomegalovirus infections of the retina. In: Schachat AP, ed: *Medical Retina* (Volume 2 of Ryan SJ, ed-in-chief: *Retina*). 3rd ed. St Louis: CV Mosby Co; 2001;1558–1575.

Cunningham ET Jr, Short GA, Irvine AR, et al: Acquired immunodeficiency syndrome–associated herpes simplex virus retinitis: clinical description and use of a polymerase chain reaction–based assay as a diagnostic tool. *Arch Ophthalmol* 1996;114:834–840.

Curi AL, Muralha A, Muralha L, et al: Suspension of anticytomegalovirus maintenance therapy following immune recovery due to highly active antiretroviral therapy. *Br J Ophthalmol* 2001;85:471–473.

Davis JL: Differential diagnosis of CMV retinitis. *Ocul Immunol Inflamm* 1999;7:159–166.

Eid Farah M, Muccioli C, Rinkevicius M, et al: Cystoid macular edema in patients with acquired immune deficiency syndrome and cytomegalovirus retinitis. *Eur J Ophthalmol* 2000;10:233–238.

Engstrom RE Jr, Holland GN, Hardy WD, et al: Hemorheologic abnormalities in patients with human immunodeficiency virus infection and ophthalmic microvasculopathy. *Am J Ophthalmol* 1990;109:153–161.

Font RL, Laucirica R, Patrinely JR: Immunoblastic B-cell malignant lymphoma involving the orbit and maxillary sinus in a patient with acquired immune deficiency syndrome. *Ophthalmology* 1993;100:966–970.

Freeman WR, Chen A, Henderly DE, et al: Prevalence and significance of acquired immunodeficiency syndrome–related retinal microvasculopathy. *Am J Ophthalmol* 1989;107:229–235.

Fujikawa LS, Schwartz LK, Rosenbaum EH: Acquired immunodeficiency·syndrome associated with Burkitt's lymphoma presenting with ocular findings. *Ophthalmology* 1983;90(suppl):50.

Glasgow BJ, Weisberger AK: A quantitative and cartographic study of retinal microvasculopathy in acquired immunodeficiency syndrome. *Am J Ophthalmol* 1994;118:46–56.

Gonzalez CR, Wiley CA, Arevalo JF, et al: Polymerase chain reaction detection of cytomegalovirus and human immunodeficiency virus-1 in the retina of patients with acquired immune deficiency syndrome with and without cotton-wool spots. *Retina* 1996;16:305–311.

Henderson HW, Mitchell SM: Treatment of immune recovery vitritis with local steroids. *Br J Ophthalmol* 1999;83:540–545.

Herbort CP, LeHoang P: Cytomegalovirus retinitis in AIDS patients: 1999 update. *Ocul Immunol Inflamm* 1999;7:123–128.

Holland GN: Immune recovery uveitis. *Ocul Immunol Inflamm* 1999;7:215–221.

Holland GN: New issues in the management of patients with AIDS-related cytomegalovirus retinitis. *Arch Ophthalmol* 2000;118:704–706.

Holland GN: New strategies for the management of AIDS-related CMV retinitis in the era of potent antiretroviral therapy. *Ocul Immunol Inflamm* 1999;7:179–188.

Iragui VJ, Kalmijn J, Plummer DJ, et al: Pattern electroretinograms and visual evoked potentials in HIV infection: evidence of asymptomatic retinal and postretinal impairment in the absence of infectious retinopathy. *Neurology* 1996;47:1452–1456.

Jabs DA: Discontinuing anticytomegalovirus therapy in patients with cytomegalovirus retinitis and AIDS. *Br J Ophthalmol* 2001;85:381–382.

Jacobson MA: Treatment of cytomegalovirus retinitis in patients with the acquired immunodeficiency syndrome. *N Engl J Med* 1997;337:105–114.

Jacobson MA, Schrier R, McCune JM, et al: Cytomegalovirus (CMV)–specific CD4$^+$ T lymphocyte immune function in long-term survivors of AIDS-related CMV end-organ disease who are receiving potent antiretroviral therapy. *J Infect Dis* 2001;183:1399–1404.

Jacobson MA, Stanley H, Holtzer C, et al: Natural history and outcome of new AIDS-related cytomegalovirus retinitis diagnosed in the era of highly active antiretroviral therapy. *Clin Infect Dis* 2000;30:231–233.

Jalali S, Reed JB, Mizoguchi M, et al: Effect of highly active antiretroviral therapy on the incidence of HIV-related cytomegalovirus retinitis and retinal detachment. *AIDS Patient Care STDS* 2000;14:343–346.

Jouan M, Saves M, Tubiana R, et al: Discontinuation of maintenance therapy for cytomegalovirus retinitis in HIV-infected patients receiving highly active antiretroviral therapy. *AIDS* 2001; 15:23–31.

Karavellas MP, Azen SP, MacDonald JC, et al: Immune recovery vitritis and uveitis in AIDS: clinical predictors, sequelae, and treatment outcomes. *Retina* 2001;21:1–9.

Karavellas MP, Lowder CY, Macdonald C, et al: Immune recovery vitritis associated with inactive cytomegalovirus retinitis: a new syndrome. *Arch Ophthalmol* 1998;116:169–175.

Karavellas MP, Plummer DJ, Macdonald JC, et al: Incidence of immune recovery vitritis in cytomegalovirus retinitis patients following institution of successful highly active antiretroviral therapy. *J Infect Dis* 1999;179:697–700.

Karavellas MP, Song M, Macdonald JC, et al: Long-term posterior and anterior segment complications of immune recovery uveitis associated with cytomegalovirus retinitis. *Am J Ophthalmol* 2000;130:57–64.

Kempen JH, Jabs DA, Dunn JP, et al: Retinal detachment risk in cytomegalovirus retinitis related to the acquired immunodeficiency syndrome. *Arch Ophthalmol* 2001;119:33–40.

Kestelyn P, Taelman H, Bogaerts J, et al: Ophthalmic manifestations of infection with *Cryptococcus neoformans* in patients with the acquired immunodeficiency syndrome. *Am J Ophthalmol* 1993;116:721–727.

Komanduri KV, Feinberg J, Hutchins RK, et al: Loss of cytomegalovirus-specific CD4+ T cell responses in human immunodeficiency virus type 1–infected patients with high CD4+ T cell counts and recurrent retinitis. *J Infect Dis* 2001; 183:1285–1289.

Kuppermann BD, Holland GN: Immune recovery uveitis. *Am J Ophthalmol* 2000;130:103–106.

Latkany PA, Holopigian K, Lorenzo-Latkany M, et al: Electroretinographic and psychophysical findings during early and late stages of human immunodeficiency virus infection and cytomegalovirus retinitis. *Ophthalmology* 1997;104:445–453.

Macdonald JC, Karavellas MP, Torriani FJ, et al: Highly active antiretroviral therapy–related immune recovery in AIDS patients with cytomegalovirus retinitis. *Ophthalmology* 2000;107:877–881.

Matzkin DC, Slamovits TL, Rosenbaum PS: Simultaneous intraocular and orbital non-Hodgkin lymphoma in the acquired immune deficiency syndrome. *Ophthalmology* 1994;101:850–855.

Mittra RA, Pulido JS, Hanson GA, et al: Primary ocular Epstein-Barr virus–associated non-Hodgkin's lymphoma in a patient with AIDS: a clinicopathologic report. *Retina* 1999;19:45–50.

Moorthy RS, Weinberg DV, Teich SA, et al: Management of varicella zoster virus retinitis in AIDS. *Br J Ophthalmol* 1997;81:189–194.

Nguyen QD, Kempen JH, Bolton SG, et al: Immune recovery uveitis in patients with AIDS and cytomegalovirus retinitis after highly active antiretroviral therapy. *Am J Ophthalmol* 2000;129: 634–639.

Nussenblatt RB, Lane HC: Human immunodeficiency virus disease: changing patterns of intraocular inflammation. *Am J Ophthalmol* 1998;125:374–382.

Ormerod LD, Puklin JE: AIDS-associated intraocular lymphoma causing primary retinal vasculitis. *Ocul Immunol Inflamm* 1997;5:271–278.

Park KL, Marx JL, Lopez PF, et al: Noninfectious branch retinal vein occlusion in HIV-positive patients. *Retina* 1997;17:162–164.

Plummer DJ, Sample PA, Arevalo JF, et al: Visual field loss in HIV-positive patients without infectious retinopathy. *Am J Ophthalmol* 1996;122:542–549.

Plummer DJ, Sample PA, Freeman WR: Visual dysfunction in HIV-positive patients without infectious retinopathy. *AIDS Patient Care STDS* 1998;12:171–179.

Postelmans L, Gerard M, Sommereijns B, et al: Discontinuation of maintenance therapy for CMV retinitis in AIDS patients on highly active antiretroviral therapy. *Ocul Immunol Inflamm* 1999;7:199–203.

Postelmans L, Payen MC, De Wit S, et al: Neovascularization of the optic disc after highly active antiretroviral therapy in an AIDS patient with cytomegalovirus retinitis: a new immune recovery–related ocular disorder? *Ocul Immunol Inflamm* 1999;7:237–240.

Quiceno JI, Capparelli E, Sadun AA, et al: Visual dysfunction without retinitis in patients with acquired immunodeficiency syndrome. *Am J Ophthalmol* 1992;113:8–13.

Raina J, Bainbridge JW, Shah SM: Decreased visual acuity in patients with cytomegalovirus retinitis and AIDS. *Eye* 2000;14:8–12.

Rao NA, Zimmerman PL, Boyer D, et al: A clinical, histopathologic, and electron microscopic study of *Pneumocystis carinii* choroiditis. *Am J Ophthalmol* 1989;107:218–228.

Robinson MR, Reed G, Csaky KG, et al: Immune-recovery uveitis in patients with cytomegalovirus retinitis taking highly active antiretroviral therapy. *Am J Ophthalmol* 2000;130:49–56.

Robinson MR, Ross ML, Whitcup SM: Ocular manifestations of HIV infection. *Curr Opin Ophthalmol* 1999;10:431–437.

Roth DB, McCabe CM, Davis JL: HIV-related occlusive vasculitis. *Arch Ophthalmol* 1999;117:696–698.

Sadun AA, Pepose JS, Madigan MC, et al: AIDS-related optic neuropathy: a histological, virological and ultrastructural study. *Graefes Arch Clin Exp Ophthalmol* 1995;233:387–398.

Saran BR, Pomilla PV: Retinal vascular nonperfusion and retinal neovascularization as a consequence of cytomegalovirus retinitis and cryptococcal choroiditis. *Retina* 1996;16:510–512.

Schanzer MC, Font RL, O'Malley RE: Primary ocular malignant lymphoma associated with the acquired immune deficiency syndrome. *Ophthalmology* 1991;98:88–91.

Shami MJ, Freeman W, Friedberg D, et al: A multicenter study of *Pneumocystis* choroidopathy. *Am J Ophthalmol* 1991;112:15–22.

Sommerhalder J, Baglivo E, Barbey C, et al: Colour vision in AIDS patients without HIV retinopathy. *Vis Res* 1998;38:3441–3446.

Song MK, Karavellas MP, MacDonald JC, et al: Characterization of reactivation of cytomegalovirus retinitis in patients healed after treatment with highly active antiretroviral therapy. *Retina* 2000;20:151–155.

Stanton CA, Sloan B III, Slusher MM, et al: Acquired immunodeficiency syndrome–related primary intraocular lymphoma. *Arch Ophthalmol* 1992;110:1614–1617.

Tenhula WN, Xu SZ, Madigan MC, et al: Morphometric comparisons of optic nerve axon loss in acquired immunodeficiency syndrome. *Am J Ophthalmol* 1992;113:14–20.

Tufail A, Holland GN, Fisher TC, et al: Increased polymorphonuclear leucocyte rigidity in HIV infected individuals. *Br J Ophthalmol* 2000;84: 727–731.

Velez G, Roy CE, Whitcup SM, et al: High-dose intravitreal ganciclovir and foscarnet for cytomegalovirus retinitis. *Am J Ophthalmol* 2001;131: 396–397.

Vrabec TR: Advances in the diagnosis and management of AIDS-related eye disease. *Curr Opin Ophthalmol* 1998;9:93–99.

Zegans M, Marsh B, Walton RC: Cytomegalovirus retinitis in the era of highly active antiretroviral therapy. *Int Ophthalmol Clin* 2000;40: 127–135.

Zegans ME, Walton RC, Holland GN, et al: Transient vitreous inflammatory reactions associated with combination antiretroviral therapy in patients with AIDS and cytomegalovirus retinitis. *Am J Ophthalmol* 1998;125:292–300.

Neuro-Ophthalmic Manifestations

Although more than 75% of HIV-positive patients show central or peripheral nervous system histopathologic changes related to their HIV disease at autopsy, only 40% to 50% of patients show neurologic symptoms during active HIV infection. In general, HIV-related neurologic disorders may be grouped as either primary, those related most directly to HIV itself, or secondary, those resulting from opportunistic infections and neoplasms. Clinical neuro-ophthalmic syndromes produced by HIV or HIV-related opportunistic disorders are discussed in this chapter. In general, both primary and secondary neurologic disorders are more common in the setting of advanced HIV disease.

7-1

PRIMARY DISORDERS

It is important to distinguish primary HIV-related headache, meningitis, and encephalopathy causing cognitive impairment and dementia from secondary opportunistic infections and neoplasms. Making these distinctions can often be quite difficult, however, and usually requires a synthesis of each patient's clinical findings, laboratory investigations, imaging studies, and cerebrospinal fluid analyses.

HIV enters the central nervous system soon after infection, where microglial cells and macrophages appear to be the primary reservoirs for both productive and latent infection. Early neurologic symptoms occur most commonly during the 3 to 4 weeks after infection and usually develop in association with a flu-like illness. Headache is particularly common, but other clinical syndromes may also occur, including focal or diffuse encephalitis or leukoencephalopathy, meningitis, ataxia, myelopathy, or peripheral neuropathy. Cerebrospinal fluid analysis performed during an acute infection is typically nonspecific. Most patients show a mild lymphocytic pleocytosis, with a modest rise in protein. The results of neuroimaging studies, if performed, are usually normal.

Neurologic symptoms can also occur during the period of latent, or clinically "asymptomatic," infection, but are less frequent. The most commonly encountered disorders include a demyelinating peripheral neuropathy, which may be painful, and a multiple sclerosis–like illness. Both tend to be subacute, with periods of relative exacerbation and remission. Systemic corticosteroids can provide some improvement in certain patients.

As the immune system weakens and patients develop AIDS, primary HIV-related neurologic symptoms become more common. The most frequently encountered primary HIV-related disorders include headache, meningitis, and diffuse encephalopathy with dementia.

7-1-1 Headache

HIV headache may occur in isolation or in combination with meningeal symptoms and signs, such as photophobia and nuchal rigidity. Whereas headache is infrequently associated with an opportunistic central nervous system infection or tumor in ambulatory HIV-positive patients with mild immune suppression, such lesions are found in a high proportion of severely immunocompromised patients who complain of headache, particularly when observed in association with cranial nerve pareses or other neurologic deficits.

7-1-2 Meningitis

HIV-related meningitis occurs both early and late following infection and can produce symptoms of headache and photophobia or signs, such as nuchal rigidity or cranial nerve palsies. Focal or generalized seizures, as well as altered mental status, may also occur. Some patients develop a particularly severe and fulminant form of diffuse meningoencephalitis that can be fatal. Cerebrospinal fluid findings tend to be nonspecific and characterized by a lymphocytic pleocytosis and mild-to-moderate elevation in protein. Neuroimaging studies performed with intravenous contrast show intense signal in the meninges and may also reveal white matter and cranial nerve root enhancement. Ventricular enlargement and widening of the cortical sulci may also be present.

7-1-3 Dementia

AIDS dementia complex, also referred to as *HIV-1–associated cognitive/motor complex* or *HIV-1–associated neurocognitive disorder*, affects most HIV-infected patients with severe CD4+ T-lymphocyte depletion and is characterized by the triad of cognitive, motor, and behavioral dysfunction. Alertness is usually unaffected. Patients often experience difficulties with concentration and memory, problems with balance, gait, or hand coordination, and, in advanced stages, bowel and bladder incontinence. At the end stage, patients become unable to ambulate, unaware of their surroundings, and vegetative. Cerebrospinal fluid changes tend to be nonspecific in patients with the

AIDS dementia complex, just as in patients with HIV-associated headache and meningitis. Neuroimaging studies usually show widespread atrophy with ventriculomegaly, widening of the cortical sulci, and a reduction in the size of the basal ganglia. Focal white matter, basal ganglia, and thalamic abnormalities can also be seen. Subtle eye abnormalities in pursuit and saccadic eye movements are often present in patients with AIDS dementia complex, but can be difficult to detect without specialized equipment.

7-2

OPPORTUNISTIC INFECTIONS

A number of opportunistic infections have been reported to affect the brain of HIV-infected patients and may produce neuro-ophthalmic complications. The most common infections are cerebral toxoplasmosis, cryptococcal meningitis, progressive multifocal leukoencephalopathy, and neurosyphilis. Other causes of meningitis and of either focal or diffuse encephalitis have also been reported in HIV-positive patients, including numerous bacterial, fungal, helminthic, protozoan, and viral infections.

7-2-1 Cerebral Toxoplasmosis

Cerebral toxoplasmosis affects up to 40% of patients with AIDS worldwide, although the prevalence varies considerably, depending to a large extent on the prevalence of latent infection in different populations. Infections are more common, for example, in France and Brazil and less common in the United States. Cerebral toxoplasmosis may occur at any CD4$^+$ cell count, but appears to increase in frequency as the number of T lymphocytes falls below 200 cells/μL. Symptoms and signs of cerebral toxoplasmosis may be either generalized or focal. Common generalized symptoms and signs include headache, confusion, fever, lethargy, and seizures. Ocular complications related to cerebral infection include papilledema, visual field defects, cranial nerve palsies, and oculomotor abnormalities.

Although toxoplasmic retinochoroiditis may occur independently of cerebral infection, a sizable proportion of HIV-infected patients with toxoplasmic retinochoroiditis also have cerebral toxoplasmosis. Neuroimaging performed with the aid of contrast typically shows one or more nodular ring-enhancing lesions, most frequently located in the cerebral hemispheres (Figure 7-1). Magnetic resonance imaging (MRI) appears to be more sensitive than computed tomography (CT) for visualizing intracranial lesions. Large lesions may produce marked edema, along with shifting of the intracranial contents. Similar findings may, however, be found in patients with a central nervous system lymphoma or an infectious abscess.

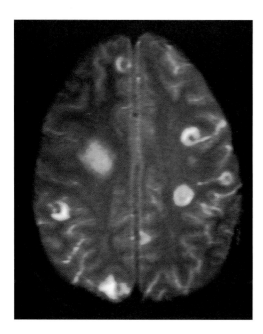

Figure 7-1 *Contrast-enhanced MRI of cerebral toxoplasmosis with classic ring lesions.*

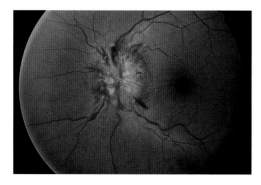

Figure 7-2 *Papilledema due to cryptococcal meningitis. Similar findings were present in fellow eye.*

The vast majority of HIV-positive patients with cerebral toxoplasmosis are immunoglobulin G (IgG)–seropositive and respond to a specific antitoxoplasmosis therapy, such as pyrimethamine and sulfadiazine, clindamycin, or atovaquone. HIV-positive patients with cerebral toxoplasmosis and a CD4+ T-lymphocyte count below 100 cells/μL require long-term antitoxoplasmosis therapy to minimize the risk of recurrences.

7-2-2 Cryptococcal Meningitis

Cryptococcal meningitis affects approximately 10% of patients with AIDS. The presenting symptoms and signs of cerebral cryptococcosis may be subtle, however, and can include fever, malaise, nausea, vomiting, and headache. Neck stiffness and photophobia are often absent. Up to 80% of HIV-positive patients with cryptococcal meningitis describe an upper respiratory illness preceding their central nervous system infection by 2 to 4 months. Papulonodular cutaneous cryptococcosis may also occur.

Neuro-ophthalmic complications affect up to 25% of HIV-positive patients with cerebral cryptococcosis. The most common findings are papilledema (Figure 7-2), which is related to increased intracranial pressure, and cryptococcal optic neuritis, which results from direct infection of the optic nerve. Cerebrospinal fluid opening pressure is elevated in the setting of papilledema, whereas it is normal in patients with disc swelling due to optic neuritis. Neuroimaging typically shows intense meningeal enhancement.

Treatment usually requires long-term use of antifungal medications, such as amphotericin B, flucytosine, or one of the azole compounds. Some patients also require intrathecal delivery of these agents to control their central nervous system infection. Recurrences are observed in up to 50% of patients.

7-2-3 Progressive Multifocal Leukoencephalopathy

Progressive multifocal leukoencephalopathy (PML) is a disorder of cerebral demyelination caused by reactivation of the JC virus, a member of the Papovaviridae family, which infects oligodendrocytes and astrocytes. PML affects less than 5% of HIV-positive patients and occurs almost exclusively at CD4+ T-lymphocyte counts less than 100 cells/μL. Presenting symptoms may include altered mental status, speech disturbances, difficulties with gait or coordination, hemiparesis, or vision loss. Seizures occur in up to 30% of patients with PML.

Visual symptoms related to involvement of the parieto-occipital cortex are common and include both homonymous visual field defects and cortical visual impairment. Disorders of ocular motility and ocular alignment may also occur. Both CT and MRI can be used to reveal characteristic white matter lesions (Figure 7-3). Definitive diagnosis may require biopsy, however. The long-term prognosis for patients with AIDS and PML is very poor.

7-2-4 Neurosyphilis

Neurosyphilis and syphilitic meningitis have been well described in HIV-positive patients. Meningeal inflammation may affect the cranial nerve roots, producing single or multiple palsies. In addition, a concurrent vasculitis can affect the medium-

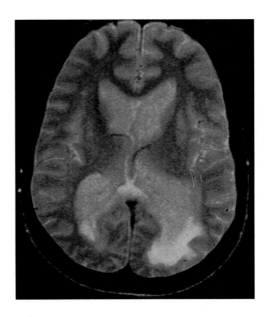

Figure 7-3 *Contrast-enhanced MRI of PML involving left occipital lobe and causing homonymous hemianopsia.*
Courtesy James P. Dunn, MD.

sized cerebral vessels that lie deep in the brain parenchyma, producing focal or multifocal deficits. Uveitis and optic disc edema are present in a sizable proportion of patients.

Diagnosis requires identification of positive syphilis serologies, which should include specific antitreponemal serum antibody testing (fluorescent treponemal antibody absorption [FTA-ABS] test or microhemagglutination assay for *Treponema pallidum* [MHA-TP]), nonspecific serum antibody testing (Venereal Disease Research Laboratory [VDRL] or rapid plasma reagin [RPR] test), and nonspecific cerebrospinal fluid testing (VDRL or RPR). While the FTA-ABS and MHA-TP tests are quite sensitive, the VDRL and RPR tests may yield false-negative results in up to 30% of HIV-infected patients. Treatment includes intravenous penicillin G, 24 million units/ day for 7 to 14 days.

7-3

OPPORTUNISTIC NEOPLASMS

Primary central nervous system lymphoma is the most common intracranial neoplasm in HIV-positive patients, affecting up to 5% of patients. CD4+ T-lymphocyte counts are typically under 50 cells/µL. Central nervous system lymphomas tend to grow slowly and may be clinically silent in up to 50% of patients. Histologically, the tumor is usually composed of both small and large B cells, most of which appear to contain Epstein-Barr virus DNA. Symptoms, when present, may include confusion, memory loss, lethargy, and headache. Focal or multifocal neurologic deficits are also common. Recognized ocular complications include progressive optic atrophy, oculomotor nerve pareses, and oculomotor abnormalities. Papilledema and visual field defects may also occur, but are less common.

Neuroimaging techniques allow for precise localization of the lesions (Figure 7-4), but definitive diagnosis usually requires stereotactic biopsy. Polymerase chain reaction–based amplification of Epstein-Barr virus DNA from cerebrospinal fluid may support the diagnosis. Long-term prognosis is generally poor, although combined use of corticosteroids and radiation therapy, with or without chemotherapy, has had limited success.

7-4

CLINICAL NEURO-OPHTHALMIC SYNDROMES

Neuro-ophthalmic manifestations occur in 10% to 15% of HIV-infected patients. The most common findings include optic nerve head edema, related to either papilledema or optic neuritis, optic atrophy, visual field defects, oculomotor nerve pareses, and oculomotor abnormalities. Virtually any infectious or neoplastic process can produce these changes, but cerebral toxoplasmosis, central nervous system lymphoma, PML, cerebral cryptococcosis, and neurosyphilis are most frequent in patients with HIV disease.

7-4-1 Papilledema

Papilledema, or optic disc swelling resulting from increased intracranial pressure, occurs in less than 5% of patients with AIDS. Patients may be asymptomatic or may have headache, with or without nausea. Cranial nerve pareses may also occur, with the sixth cranial nerve being involved most frequently. The most common causes in HIV-positive patients are cryptococcal meningitis and cerebral toxoplasmosis. Papilledema is typically bilateral, but may be asymmetric.

All patients with disc swelling should undergo contrast-enhanced neuroimaging to localize and characterize any possible intracranial lesions. If there is no mass effect or if the scan results are normal, patients should then have a lumbar puncture to measure opening cerebrospinal pressure. Other tests that should be run on the cerebrospinal fluid include cell count, protein, glucose, VDRL or RPR, India ink stain, acid-fast bacillus stain and culture, cryptococcal antigen, routine culture and sensitivity, and cytology to exclude carcinomatous or lymphomatous meningitis.

7-4-2 Optic Neuritis

The term *optic neuritis* is used most often for patients with presumed demyelinating disease who present with decreased vision, an afferent pupillary defect, and optic disc edema. In the broader sense, however, optic neuritis may be taken as any inflam-

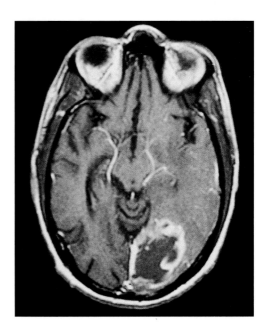

Figure 7-4 *Contrast-enhanced MRI of cerebral lymphoma involving left occipital lobe.*
Courtesy James P. Dunn, MD.

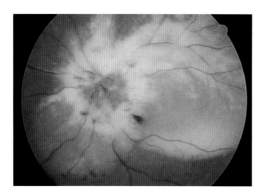

Figure 7-5 *CMV papillitis producing peripapillary and macular serous retinal detachment.*

Reproduced with permission of the publisher from Cunningham ET Jr, Pepose JS, Holland GN: Cytomegalovirus infections of the retina. In: Schachat AP, ed: Medical Retina *(Volume 2 of Ryan SJ, ed-in-chief:* Retina*). 3rd ed. St Louis: CV Mosby Co; 2001;1558–1575.*

matory or infectious process that produces these symptoms and signs. An alternate term for inflammatory or infectious disc swelling is *papillitis.*

Perhaps the most common cause of optic disc edema in HIV-positive patients is cytomegalovirus (CMV) papillitis, which affects 5% to 10% of HIV-positive patients and may be associated with a peripapillary or macular serous retinal detachment (Figure 7-5). As with CMV retinitis, CMV papillitis occurs most often at CD4$^+$ T-lymphocyte counts below 100 cells/μL. While CMV papillitis responds to standard CMV therapy (see Chapter 6, "Posterior Segment Manifestations"), prolonged induction times of 3 to 6 weeks with anti-CMV therapy have been recommended.

Other causes of papillitis believed to be more common in HIV-infected patients include syphilis, cryptococcosis, herpes simplex virus infection, varicella zoster virus infection, toxoplasmosis, tuberculosis, and lymphoma (Figure 7-6). Didanosine (2′,3′-dideoxyinosine), a nucleoside analog used to treat HIV infection, has been reported to cause optic neuritis in an isolated case of a 40-year-old HIV-positive man with a CD4$^+$ T-lymphocyte count of 190 cells/μL.

7-4-3 Optic Atrophy

HIV-positive patients may develop a painless, progressive atrophy of the optic nerve associated with loss of color vision, decreased contrast sensitivity, and visual field defects. The cause of HIV-related optic neuropathy is unknown, but these symptoms may represent the cumulative damage of ongoing HIV retinopathy. All patients with optic disc pallor should, however, be evaluated for the possible presence of retro-bulbar or intracranial infection or tumor. Systemic medications, such as ethambutol, which is used to treat tuberculosis, can also cause a progressive optic atrophy and should be considered in patients receiving such treatments.

7-4-4 Visual Field Defects and Cortical Vision Loss

Visual field defects may result from any insult to the retrobulbar visual pathways. Homonymous visual field defects are particularly common in patients with cerebral toxoplasmosis and PML (see Figure 7-3). Large lesions involving the optic radiations or the occipital cortex may cause cortical vision loss or even cortical blindness, a syndrome that affects 5% to 10% of patients with PML at the time of their initial diagnosis. Chiasmal syndromes may also occur, but are infrequent. In general, visual field defects are less common in the setting of primary central nervous system lymphoma or in patients with infectious or tumor-related meningitis, but can occur when there is extensive involvement of the meninges overlying the visual cortex.

7-4-5 Oculomotor Nerve Paresis

Partial or complete paresis of one or more of the oculomotor nerves may occur as a result of either parenchymal or meningeal disease. Common causes in HIV-infected patients include cerebral toxoplasmosis and basal meningitis in the setting of cryptococcosis, syphilis, or tuberculosis. Sixth-nerve involvement is particularly common and

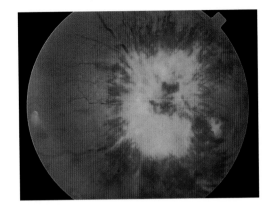

Figure 7-6 *Intraocular lymphoma presenting as severe papillitis.*
Courtesy Cristina Muccioli, MD.

usually results from increased intracranial pressure. The mass effect of primary central nervous system lymphomas may also produce isolated or multiple oculomotor nerve palsies, but cranial nerve pareses are more common in patients with lymphomatous meningitis, which most often results from metastatic spread of systemic lymphoma. HIV-positive patients who develop an oculomotor nerve paresis should undergo contrast-enhanced neuroimaging and a lumbar puncture to measure opening pressure and provide cerebrospinal fluid for analysis, as outlined above.

7-4-6 Oculomotor Disorders

HIV-related infections and tumors may cause a number of well-recognized oculomotor disorders, including internuclear ophthalmoplegia, horizontal and vertical gaze pareses, the dorsal midbrain (or Parinaud) syndrome, nystagmus, and skew deviation. The approach to diagnosis in HIV-positive patients with oculomotor abnormalities is essentially the same as that described above for patients with cranial nerve pareses.

SELECTED REFERENCES

Bacellar H, Munoz A, Miller EN, et al: Temporal trends in the incidence of HIV-1–related neurologic diseases. Multicenter AIDS Cohort Study, 1985–1992. *Neurology* 1994;44:1892–1900.

Berger JR, Major EO: Progressive multifocal leukoencephalopathy. *Sem Neurol* 1999;19: 193–200.

Cohen BA: Neurologic manifestations of toxoplasmosis in AIDS. *Sem Neurol* 1999;19:201–211.

Cunningham ET Jr, Pepose JS, Holland GN: Cytomegalovirus infections of the retina. In: Schachat AP, ed: *Medical Retina* (Volume 2 of Ryan SJ, ed-in-chief: *Retina*). 3rd ed. St. Louis: CV Mosby Co; 2001;1558–1575.

Currie J: AIDS and neuro-ophthalmology. *Curr Opin Ophthalmol* 1995;6:34–40.

Currie J, Dwyer E: Retroviruses and the acquired immune deficiency syndrome. In: Miller NR, Newman NJ, eds: *Walsh and Hoyt's Clinical Neuro-Ophthalmology.* 5th ed. Baltimore, MD: Williams & Wilkins; 1998;5:5361–5464.

Friedman DI: Neuro-ophthalmic manifestations of human immunodeficiency virus infection. *Neurol Clin* 1991;9:55–72.

Hamed LM, Schatz NJ, Galetta SL: Brainstem ocular motility defects and AIDS. *Am J Ophthalmol* 1988;106:437–442.

Hedges TR III: Ophthalmoplegia associated with AIDS. *Surv Ophthalmol* 1994;39:43–51.

Keane JR: Neuro-ophthalmologic signs of AIDS: 50 patients. *Neurology* 1991;41:841–845.

Mansour AM: Neuro-ophthalmic findings in acquired immunodeficiency syndrome. *J Clin Neuroophthalmol* 1990;10:167–174.

Nichols JW, Goodwin JA: Neuro-ophthalmologic complications of AIDS. *Sem Ophthalmol* 1992;7: 24–29.

Price RW: Management of the neurologic complications of HIV-1 infection and AIDS. In: Sande MA, Volberding PA, eds: *The Medical Management of AIDS*. 6th ed. Philadelphia: WB Saunders Co; 1999:217–240.

Quiceno JI, Capparelli E, Sadun AA, et al: Visual dysfunction without retinitis in patients with acquired immunodeficiency syndrome. *Am J Ophthalmol* 1992;113:8–13.

Tardieu M: HIV-1–related central nervous system diseases. *Curr Opin Neurol* 1999;12:377–381.

Warren FA: Neuroophthalmologic and orbital manifestations of AIDS. In: Stenson SM, Friedberg DN, eds: *AIDS and the Eye*. New Orleans: Contact Lens Association of Ophthalmologists; 1995:107–123.

Winward KE, Hamed LM, Glaser JS: The spectrum of optic nerve disease in human immunodeficiency virus infection. *Am J Ophthalmol* 1989; 107:373–380.

Yen MY: Neuro-ophthalmologic manifestations of systemic disease. *Curr Opin Ophthalmol* 1992; 3:592–598.

CHAPTER 8

Manifestations in Children

More than 1 million of the world's children are currently infected with HIV. Most HIV-positive children acquired their infection perinatally, either in utero, at delivery, or while breast-feeding. In the absence of specific antiretroviral treatment, mother-to-child transmission of HIV occurs in up to one third of deliveries. Not unexpectedly, therefore, the prevalence of HIV positivity among children generally parallels the infection rate in pregnant women around the world, with more than 90% of all HIV-positive children living in Africa. In the United States, more than half of all children with HIV live in New York, Florida, California, or Puerto Rico. In Europe, roughly 60% of all reported pediatric AIDS patients live in Romania. While the number of children born with HIV has been decreasing in industrialized countries each year, due in large part to the aggressive use of perinatal antiretroviral agents, the number of children born with HIV continues to increase in developing countries.

8-1

AIDS DEFINITION IN CHILDREN

Children normally have much higher CD4+ T-lymphocyte counts than do adults. For this reason, both the Centers for Disease Control and Prevention (CDC) and the World Health Organization (WHO) have modified their AIDS-defining CD4+ T-lymphocyte levels as less than 750 cells/µL for children under 1 year of age and as less than 500 cells/µL for children 1 to 5 years of age. The same AIDS-defining CD4+ count used for adults, less than 200 cells/µL, is used for all children 6 years of age and older.

8-2

SEROLOGIC TESTING

Serologic testing for HIV infection in newborns can be complicated by the presence of maternal anti-HIV antibodies, which can persist for months in the newborn. For this reason, direct viral detection techniques, such as HIV DNA or RNA levels performed on peripheral blood mononuclear cells, are used most often during this period. Viral detection techniques are less sensitive, however, during the first few weeks of life.

TABLE 8-1

Centers for Disease Control and Prevention 1994 Revised HIV Pediatric Classification System: Immune Categories Based on Age-Specific CD4⁺ T-Lymphocyte Count and Percent

Immune Category	CD4⁺ T-Lymphocyte Count, cells/µL (%)		
	<12 Months	**1–5 Years**	**6–12 Years**
1: No suppression	>1500 (>25%)	>1000 (>25%)	>500 (>25%)
2: Moderate suppression	750–1499 (15%–24%)	500–999 (15%–24%)	200–499 (15%–24%)
3: Severe suppression	<750 (<15%)	<500 (<15%)	<200 (<15%)

8-3

CLINICAL CHARACTERISTICS

HIV infection is more aggressive in children than in adults, usually producing symptoms within the first year of life. The median survival time for HIV-infected children prior to the advent of highly active antiretroviral therapy (HAART) ranged from 5 to 8 years, significantly less than the median survival time of approximately 10 years in adults. Of note, HIV-infected children tend to have persistently high viral loads, perhaps due to the inability of their relatively immature immune systems to establish an effective cytotoxic T-lymphocyte response to HIV.

Recurrent bacterial infections are more common in HIV-infected children than in adults with HIV disease. Common causes of bacteremia include *Streptococcus pneumoniae, Haemophilus influenzae,* and *Salmonella* species, whereas genitourinary tract infections are typically due to *Escherichia coli,* and skin and soft tissue diseases are commonly caused by *Staphylococcus aureus* and *Streptococcus viridans.* Other clinical syndromes encountered in HIV-positive children include sinusitis, pneumonia, osteomyelitis, septic arthritis, otitis media, and meningitis.

CD4⁺ cell counts remain a good predictor of risk for opportunistic disorders in HIV-positive children, but must be age-corrected. The CDC has published age-specific ranges for three immune categories based on CD4⁺ cell counts in children; the categories are numbered 1, 2, and 3, respectively (Table 8-1):

1: No suppression
2: Moderate suppression
3: Severe suppression

Clinical categories, which reflect signs and symptoms in HIV-infected children, have also been created (Table 8-2):

N: None
A: Mild
B: Moderate
C: Severe

TABLE 8-2

Centers for Disease Control and Prevention 1994 Revised HIV Pediatric Classification System: Clinical Categories Based on Signs and Symptoms

Clinical Category	Diagnosis
N: None	Asymptomatic; single category A event

A: Mild	Mildly symptomatic, with two or more of the following:
	    dermatitis
	    hepatomegaly
	    lymphadenopathy
	    parotitis
	    recurrent upper respiratory tract infection, sinusitis, or otitis media
	    splenomegaly

B: Moderate	Moderately symptomatic, with one or more of the following:
	    anemia
	    cardiomyopathy
	    cytomegalovirus (CMV) infection at <1 month of age
	    hepatitis
	    lymphoid interstitial pneumonia
	    neutropenia
	    pneumonia
	    thrombocytopenia

C: Severe	Severely symptomatic, with one or more of the following:
	    Burkitt or immunoblastic lymphoma
	    cryptosporidiosis or isosporiasis
	    cytomegalovirus (CMV) disease at >1 month of age
	    disseminated coccidioidomycosis
	    disseminated histoplasmosis
	    disseminated *Mycobacterium avium*
	    disseminated or extrapulmonary mycobacterial tuberculosis
	    disseminated other or unspecified *Mycobacteria* species
	    encephalopathy
	    esophageal or pulmonary candidiasis
	    extrapulmonary cryptococcosis
	    herpes simplex virus (HSV) infection at >1 month of age
	    Kaposi sarcoma
	    multiple recurrent severe bacterial infections
	    Pneumocystis carinii pneumonia
	    primary lymphoma of brain
	    progressive multifocal leukoencephalopathy (PML)
	    recurrent *Salmonella* (nontyphoid) septicemia
	    toxoplasmosis of brain at >1 month of age
	    wasting syndrome

For example, a child categorized as A2 is mildly symptomatic and moderately immune-suppressed, whereas a child categorized as N3 is asymptomatic, but severely immune-suppressed. Predictors of rapid disease progression in children include early infection, early onset of HIV-related conditions, failure to thrive, generalized lymphadenopathy, and high viral loads after 1 month of life.

8-4

OCULAR COMPLICATIONS

8-4-1 Cytomegalovirus Retinitis

Cytomegalovirus (CMV) retinitis is the most commonly encountered ocular complication of HIV/AIDS in children. Any aspect of the fundus may be involved, including the optic disc (Figure 8-1). Relevant studies are summarized below:

1. Dennehy and associates examined 40 HIV-positive children in Miami, Florida, over a 2-year period between 1986 and 1988. All of the children had been infected perinatally. Only 2 children (5%) developed CMV retinitis.

2. De Smet and colleagues, at the National Eye Institute (NEI), described their cohort of HIV-infected children in both 1992 and 1994. Overall, 1% to 2% of the children seen during that time had CMV retinitis, although the prevalence increased to nearly 20% among the subgroup of HIV-positive children who had a $CD4^+$ T-lymphocyte count below 100 cells/µL. Of note, more than one third of the pediatric patients who had CMV retinitis went on to develop a retinal detachment.

3. Hammond and colleagues described their experience with 12 children referred with symptomatic HIV disease from a cohort of 98 HIV-positive children seen in London in 1996. All had acquired HIV disease from their mothers. Of the 12 children, 3 were found to have CMV retinitis (3.1% of the 98) and 1 had herpetic necrotizing retinitis that progressed rapidly (1%). The $CD4^+$ T-lymphocyte counts of the children with CMV retinitis ranged from 13 cells/µL to 60 cells/µL. The $CD4^+$ T-lymphocyte count of the child with herpetic necrotizing retinitis was 294 cells/µL.

4. Girard and colleagues examined 33 HIV-positive children in France in the mid-1990s, of whom 23 had AIDS. Toxoplasmic retinochoroiditis was the most common finding, and CMV retinitis was not identified.

5. Baumal and associates observed 1 child with CMV retinitis in a cohort of 17 pediatric patients with AIDS (5.9%) seen at the Hospital for Sick Children in Toronto between 1985 and 1994. The Toronto group subsequently identified 2 additional HIV-positive children with CMV retinitis in 1995 and noted that all 3 of these patients had a $CD4^+$ cell count below the fifth percentile for their age and that 2 of the 3 had bilateral disease at the time of diagnosis.

6. Walton and colleagues also described bilateral CMV retinitis at initial examination in 3 young children and suggested that aggressive combination antiviral therapy might be indicated in these patients.

7. Multicenter AIDS surveillance data would seem to suggest an overall prevalence of CMV retinitis of 2% to 4% in HIV-infected children in the United States.

The reason for the manifold lower prevalence of CMV retinitis in children as compared to adults is unknown. Most authors believe that the lower prevalence may simply reflect lower rates of CMV seropositivity in children. Others, by contrast, suggest that CMV retinitis is more easily missed in young preverbal children and may be underdiagnosed. As in adults, CMV retinitis appears to be more common in children with low CD4⁺ T-lymphocyte counts and high viral loads.

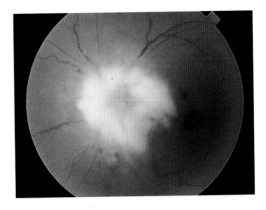

Figure 8-1 *CMV papillitis in child.*

8-4-2 Other Ocular Complications

Ocular complications of HIV infection, other than CMV retinitis, that have been reported in children include HIV retinopathy, toxoplasmic retinochoroiditis, varicella zoster virus retinitis, cutaneous molluscum contagiosum, herpes zoster ophthalmicus, keratoconjunctivitis sicca, and preseptal cellulitis. HIV-infected children also have a particularly wide range of central nervous system manifestations, including cognitive and motor deficits, impaired brain growth, and neurodevelopmental delay. Nystagmus and strabismus related to HIV encephalopathy are particularly common, as are abnormal eye movements, including abnormal pursuit, saccades, and vestibulo-ocular reflexes. Central nervous system imaging studies often reveal ventriculomegaly, cerebral atrophy, and attenuation of white matter. Calcification of the basal ganglia and white matter of the frontal lobes may also be present.

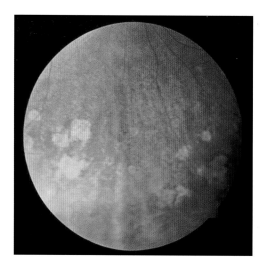

Figure 8-2 *Focal abnormalities of peripheral retinal pigment epithelium in child taking didanosine. Courtesy Scott M. Whitcup, MD.*

A fetal AIDS syndrome–associated embryopathy, including microcephaly, a prominent forehead, a flat nasal bridge, hypertelorism, mild upward or downward obliquity of the eyes, long palpebral fissures, and blue sclerae, was reported in the late 1980s, but has not been noted by subsequent investigators and appears not to be common.

8-4-3 Ocular Drug Toxicity

Ocular drug toxicity can also occur in HIV-infected children. Focal abnormalities of the peripheral retinal pigment epithelium (Figure 8-2), accompanied by abnormal electroretinography and/or electro-oculography, have been described in 5% to 10% of children taking high doses of didanosine (2′,3′-dideoxyinosine). This effect was related to both the cumulative and the peak dosages. The electrophysiologic abnormalities appeared to be reversible. Similar findings have not been observed in adults taking this medication. Stellate peripheral corneal endothelial deposits have been described in up to 25% of HIV-positive children receiving rifabutin prophylaxis for *Mycobacterium avium* complex bacteremia.

8-5

OPHTHALMIC SCREENING EXAMINATIONS

The timing and frequency of ophthalmologic examinations have not been established for children infected with HIV. Most authorities recommend a complete eye examination by 1 year of age. More frequent examinations, perhaps every 3 to 4 months, should be performed after one of the following has occurred:

1. CMV is cultured from the blood, urine, or nasopharynx

2. Nonocular end-organ CMV infection develops

3. Some other advanced HIV disease develops

4. The CD4$^+$ cell count falls below immune category 3, severe suppression (see Table 8-1)

Although most young HIV-positive children with CMV retinitis show no overt evidence of eye disease, its presence may be suggested in some patients by the presence of strabismus or visual inattention. Children with visual symptoms or signs should, of course, be examined promptly.

SELECTED REFERENCES

Abrams EJ: Opportunistic infections and other clinical manifestations of HIV disease in children. *Pediatr Clin North Am* 2000;47:79–108.

Abuzaitoun OR, Hanson IC: Organ-specific manifestations of HIV disease in children. *Pediatr Clin North Am* 2000;47:109–125.

Baumal CR, Levin AV, Kavalec CC, et al: Screening for cytomegalovirus retinitis in children. *Arch Pediatr Adolesc Med* 1996;150:1186–1192.

Baumal CR, Levin AV, Read SE: Cytomegalovirus retinitis in immunosuppressed children. *Am J Ophthalmol* 1999;127:550–558.

Biswas J, Kumar AA, George AE, et al: Ocular and systemic lesions in children with HIV. *Indian J Pediatr* 2000;67:721–724.

Bottoni F, Gonnella P, Autelino A, et al: Diffuse necrotizing retinochoroiditis in a child with AIDS and toxoplasmic encephalitis. *Graefes Arch Clin Exp Ophthalmol* 1989;84:683–687.

Bremond-Gignac D, Aron-Rosa D, Rohrlich P, et al: [Cytomegalovirus retinitis in children with AIDS acquired through materno-fetal transmission.] *J Fr Ophtalmol* 1995;18:91–95.

Centers for Disease Control and Prevention: 1994 revised classification system for human immunodeficiency virus infection in children less than 13 years of age. *MMWR* 1994;43(RR-12):1.

Cervia J: HIV/AIDS rounds: HIV in children. *AIDS Patient Care STDS.* 1999;13:165–173.

Chandwani S, Kaul A, Bebenroth D, et al: Cytomegalovirus infection in human immunodeficiency virus type 1–infected children. *Pediatr Infect Dis J* 1996;15:310–314.

Constantinescu AF, Ruta SM, Constantinescu SN, et al: Neuroophthalmological examination in children with AIDS. *Rev Roumaine Virol* 1993; 44:187–193.

Coulter JB: HIV infection in children: the widening gap between developing and industrialized countries. *Ann Trop Paediatr* 1998;18(suppl): S15–S20.

Dennehy PJ, Warman R, Flynn JT, et al: Ocular manifestations in pediatric patients with acquired immunodeficiency syndrome. *Arch Ophthalmol* 1989;107:978–982.

De Smet MD, Butler KM, Rubin BI, et al: The ocular complications of HIV in the pediatric population. In: Dernouchamps JP, Verougstraete C, Caspers-Velu L, et al, eds: *Recent Advances in Uveitis: Proceedings of the Third International Symposium on Uveitis.* Brussels, Belgium, May 24–27, 1992. Amsterdam: Kugler Publications; 1993: 315-319.

De Smet MD, Nussenblatt RB: Ocular manifestations of HIV in the pediatric population. In: Pizzo PA, Wilfert CM, eds: *Pediatric AIDS: The Challenge of HIV Infection in Infants, Children and Adolescents.* 2nd ed. Baltimore, MD: Williams & Wilkins; 1994:457–466.

Englund JA, Baker CJ, Raskino C, et al: Clinical and laboratory characteristics of a large cohort of symptomatic, human immunodeficiency virus–infected infants and children. *Pediatr Infect Dis J* 1996;15:1025–1036.

European Centre for the Epidemiological Monitoring of AIDS: European case definition for AIDS surveillance in children: revision 1995. *HIV/AIDS Surveillance in Europe.* Quarterly Report. 1995;48:46–53.

Frenkel LD, Gaur S, Tsolia M, et al: Cytomegalovirus infection in children with AIDS. *Rev Infect Dis* 1990;12(suppl 7):S820–S826.

Girard B, Prevost-Moravia G, Courpotin C, et al: [Ophthalmologic manifestations observed in a pediatric HIV-seropositive population.] *J Fr Ophtalmol* 1997;20:49–60.

Hammond CJ, Evans JA, Shah SM, et al: The spectrum of eye disease in children with AIDS due to vertically transmitted HIV disease: clinical findings, virology and recommendations for surveillance. *Graefes Arch Clin Exp Ophthalmol* 1997;235:125–129.

Iordanescu C, Matusa R, Denislam D, et al: [The ocular manifestations of AIDS in children.] *Oftalmologia* 1993;37:308–314.

Kestelyn P, Lepage P, Van de Perre P: Perivasculitis of the retinal vessels as an important sign in children with AIDS-related complex. *Am J Ophthalmol* 1985;100:614–615.

Kitchen BJ, Engler HD, Gill VJ, et al: Cytomegalovirus infection in children with human immunodeficiency virus infection. *Pediatr Infect Dis J* 1997;16:358–363.

Levin AV, Zeichner S, Duker JS, et al: Cytomegalovirus retinitis in an infant with acquired immunodeficiency syndrome. *Pediatrics* 1989;84:683–687.

Lindegren ML, Steinberg S, Byers RH Jr: Epidemiology of HIV/AIDS in children. *Pediatr Clin North Am* 2000;47:1–20.

Marion RW, Wiznia AA, Hutcheon RG, et al: Craniofacial dysmorphism in children with human immunodeficiency virus infection. *J Pediatr* 1988;113:784–785.

Marion RW, Wiznia AA, Hutcheon RG, et al: Fetal AIDS syndrome score: correlation between severity of dysmorphism and age at diagnosis of immunodeficiency. *Am J Dis Child* 1987;141:429–431.

Marion RW, Wiznia AA, Hutcheon RG, et al: Human T-cell lymphotropic virus type III (HTLV-III) embryopathy: a new dysmorphic syndrome associated with intrauterine HTLV-III infection. *Am J Dis Child* 1986;140:638–640.

Marum LH, Tindyebwa D, Gibb D: Care of children with HIV infection and AIDS in Africa. *AIDS* 1997;11(suppl B):S125–S134.

Melvin AJ, Frenkel LM: Pediatric human immunodeficiency virus type 1 infection: updates on prevention and management. *AIDS Clin Rev* 2000–2001:63–83.

Melvin AJ, Rodrigo AG, Mohan KM, et al: HIV-1 dynamics in children. *J Acquired Immune Defic Syndromes Hum Retrovirol* 1999;20:468–473.

Nicholas SW: The opportunistic and bacterial infections associated with pediatric human immunodeficiency virus disease. *Acta Paediatr Suppl* 1994;400:46–50.

Nielsen K, Bryson YJ: Diagnosis of HIV infection in children. *Pediatr Clin North Am* 2000;47: 39–63.

O'Hara MA, Raphael SA, Nelson LB: Isolated anterior uveitis in a child with acquired immunodeficiency syndrome. *Ann Ophthalmol* 1991;23: 71–73.

Ojukwu IC, Epstein LG: Neurologic manifestations of infection with HIV. *Pediatr Infect Dis J* 1998;17:343–344.

Padhani DH, Manji KP, Mtanda AT: Ocular manifestations in children with HIV infection in Dar es Salaam, Tanzania. *J Trop Pediatr* 2000;46: 145–148.

Pavia AT, Christenson JC: Pediatric AIDS. In: Sande MA, Volberding PA, eds: *The Medical Management of AIDS.* 6th ed. Philadelphia: WB Saunders Co; 1999:525–535.

Rosecan LR, Laskin OL, Kalman CM, et al: Antiviral therapy with ganciclovir for cytomegalovirus retinitis and bilateral exudative retinal detachments in an immunocompromised child. *Ophthalmology* 1986;93:1401–1407.

Salvador F, Blanco R, Colin A, et al: Cytomegalovirus retinitis in pediatric acquired immunodeficiency syndrome: report of two cases. *J Pediatr Ophthalmol Strabismus* 1993;30:159–162.

Smith JA, Mueller BU, Nussenblatt RB, et al: Corneal endothelial deposits in children positive for human immunodeficiency virus receiving rifabutin prophylaxis for *Mycobacterium avium* complex bacteremia. *Am J Ophthalmol* 1999;127: 164–169.

Spira R, Lepage P, Msellati P, et al: Natural history of human immunodeficiency virus type 1 infection in children: a five-year prospective study in Rwanda. Mother-to-Child HIV-1 Transmission Study Group. *Pediatrics* 1999;104:e56.

Tejada P, Sarmiento B, Ramos JR: Retinal microvasculopathy in human immunodeficiency type 1 (HIV)–infected children. *Int Ophthalmol* 1997–1998;21:319–321.

Walton RC, Whitcup SM, Mueller BU, et al: Combined intravenous ganciclovir and foscarnet for children with recurrent cytomegalovirus retinitis. *Ophthalmology* 1995;102:1865–1870.

Whitcup SM, Butler KM, Caruso R, et al: Retinal toxicity in human immunodeficiency virus–infected children treated with 2′,3′-dideoxyinosine. *Am J Ophthalmol* 1992;113:1–7.

Whitcup SM, Dastgheib K, Nussenblatt RB, et al: A clinicopathologic report of the retinal lesions associated with didanosine. *Arch Ophthalmol* 1994;112:1594–1598.

Wilfert CM, McKinney RE Jr: When children harbor HIV. *Sci Am* 1998;279:94–95.

Zuckerman GB, Sanchez JL, Conway EE Jr: Neurologic complications of HIV infections in children. *Pediatr Ann* 1998;27:635–639.

CHAPTER 9

Manifestations in the Developing World

Most HIV-infected patients live in the developing world, yet relatively little is known about the ocular complications of HIV/AIDS in these countries. The few reports of the effects of HIV/AIDS on the eye that have appeared suggest, however, that both the patient demographics and the prevalence of opportunistic disorders vary from region to region.

The reasons for such global differences are complex. On the one hand, differences in patient demographics appear to reflect the primary route of transmission of HIV. In North America and Europe, for example, homosexual transmission is most common, and most HIV-infected patients are usually male. By contrast, more women are infected in Africa, Asia, and Latin America, where heterosexual transmission is most frequent. On the other hand, differences in the prevalence of various opportunistic disorders appear to be related most directly to two factors:

1. Relatively few HIV-positive patients live long enough in many developing countries to reach the profound levels of immunosuppression required to put themselves at risk for cytomegalovirus (CMV) retinitis and HIV retinopathy, which tend to occur as the CD4$^+$ T-lymphocyte count drops below 100 cells/µL.

2. Certain infectious diseases are more common in particular regions, such as toxoplasmosis in Brazil and fungal keratitis in Africa.

Those ocular complications of HIV/AIDS that are either more common in, or relatively unique to, various geographic regions are discussed in this chapter.

AFRICA

HIV-infected patients in Africa are typically between 20 and 50 years of age and tend to have a higher socioeconomic status, like patients in North America and Europe. By contrast, HIV infection in Africa occurs primarily in heterosexuals and is more common in women than in men. Transmission between men having sex with men and among injection drug users is relatively infrequent.

The most common nonocular disorders observed in HIV-infected African patients include tuberculosis, toxoplasmosis, and nontuberculous bacterial infections, including pneumonia, sepsis, and meningitis. HIV-2 infections are relatively unique to West Africa, but it appears that the opportunistic disorders associated with HIV-2 infection are similar to those observed in patients with HIV-1 disease.

Early prevalence surveys from Africa described herpes zoster ophthalmicus (HZO) in 15% to 20% of HIV-infected patients, suggesting that HZO might be the most

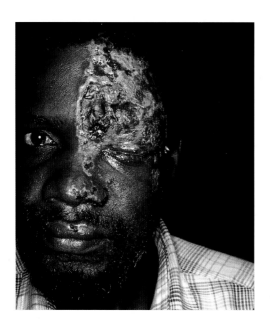

Figure 9-1 *HZO in African patient.*
Courtesy Susan Lewallen, MD.

common opportunistic infection in African patients. A 1999 study by Cochereau and colleagues in Burundi of 154 consecutive HIV-positive patients observed HZO in 1 patient, whereas a second 1999 study, by Morgan and associates in Uganda, of 105 patients infected with HIV reported no patients with HZO. These more recent data suggest that HIV-associated HZO in Africa either is less common than was previously thought or varies considerably from country to country within the continent. Regardless of prevalence in Africa, however, HZO appears to be a strong predictor of HIV infection, with more than two thirds of African patients who had HZO testing positive for HIV (Figure 9-1). Moreover, most HIV-positive patients in Africa who develop HZO go untreated, so more than 50% have or will develop a concurrent keratitis and/or uveitis. Many of these patients will, in turn, be left with markedly reduced vision.

Both CMV retinitis and HIV retinopathy occur in Africa, but are less common than in the developed world, in that they each affect less than 10% of HIV-positive patients. These numbers are lower than those reported from HIV clinics in North America and Europe, primarily because HIV-positive patients in Africa tend to die of other opportunistic disorders, such as tuberculosis or pneumococcal pneumonia, well before they reach the profound levels of immunosuppression required for HIV retinopathy and CMV retinitis to occur.

Another aspect of HIV in Africa is the finding of otherwise rare conjunctival squamous cell tumors (Figure 9-2), an observation that most probably reflects a higher prevalence of human papillomavirus infection in the African population at large. Similarly, ocular complications of tuberculosis, including uveitis, choroiditis, and phlyctenulosis, as well as fungal keratitis, occur more frequently in Africa than elsewhere. Other disorders reported to occur in African patients with AIDS include toxoplasmic retinochoroiditis, cryptococcal papilledema and choroiditis, Kaposi sarcoma, molluscum contagiosum, optic atrophy, and oculomotor paresis.

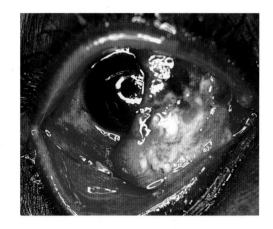

Figure 9-2 *Squamous cell tumor of conjunctiva in African patient.*
Courtesy Susan Lewallen, MD.

9-2

ASIA

A limited number of prevalence surveys have appeared from Asia:

1. Tanterdtam and colleagues described a cohort of 150 HIV-positive patients in Siriraj hospital in Thailand. Most of the patients were between 20 and 50 years of age. Cryptococcal meningitis and pulmonary tuberculosis were the most common systemic disorders, affecting approximately 9% and 5% of patients, respectively. CMV retinitis and HIV retinopathy were the most frequent ocular complications, occurring in 25% and 17%, respectively. Other ocular manifestations of HIV infection were relatively uncommon, and no patients were observed to have Kaposi sarcoma.

2. Ho and associates described 10 HIV-positive male patients in Hong Kong: 6 were homosexual, 7 had CMV retinitis, and 1 had molluscum contagiosum.

3. Biswas and colleagues described a series of 100 consecutive HIV-infected patients in Chennai, southern India. More than three fourths of the patients were men, and 70% were believed to have been infected by heterosexual transmission from commercial sex workers. Pulmonary tuberculosis was the most common systemic disorder, affecting 67% of patients. Other common sys-

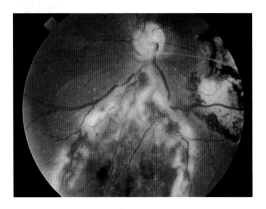

Figure 9-3 *Active CMV retinitis with adjacent toxoplasmic retinochoroidal scar in Brazilian patient. Courtesy Cristina Muccioli, MD.*

temic disorders included oropharyngeal candidiasis (66%), HIV enteropathy (16%), toxoplasmosis (15%), *Pneumocystis carinii* pneumonia (12%), and cryptococcal meningitis (5%). CMV retinitis occurred in 17% of patients, and 15% had HIV retinopathy. Only 1 patient in the cohort from Chennai had HZO, and none had Kaposi sarcoma.

9-3

LATIN AMERICA

Prevalence data from Latin America are even more limited than data from Africa and Asia. Muccioli and colleagues described a series of 445 patients from São Paulo, Brazil. More than half of the patients were homosexual men, and tuberculosis was the most common opportunistic systemic disorder, affecting 19% of patients. Ocular complications occurred in nearly 50% of patients, including CMV retinitis (25%) (Figure 9-3), toxoplasmic retinochoroiditis (9%), and non-CMV viral retinitis (4%). Other findings included papilledema (2%), optic atrophy (2%), multifocal choroiditis (1%), and syphilitic uveitis (1%).

SELECTED REFERENCES

Belfort R Jr: The ophthalmologist and the global impact of the AIDS epidemic. LV Edward Jackson Memorial Lecture. *Am J Ophthalmol* 2000; 129:1–8.

Biswas J, Madhavan HN, George AE, et al: Ocular lesions associated with HIV infection in India: a series of 100 consecutive patients evaluated at a referral center. *Am J Ophthalmol* 2000; 129:9–15.

Cochereau I, Mlika-Cabanne N, Godinaud P, et al: AIDS related eye disease in Burundi, Africa. *Br J Ophthalmol* 1999;83:339–342.

Dehne KL, Dhlakama DG, Ritcher C, et al: Herpes zoster as an indicator of HIV infection in Africa. *Trop Doctor* 1992;22:68–70.

el Matri L, Kammoun M, Cheour M, et al: [Eye involvement in AIDS: the first 12 Tunisian cases.] *Tunis Med* 1992;70:481–484.

Ho PC, Farzavandi SK, Kwok SK, et al: Ophthalmic complications of AIDS in Hong Kong. *J Hong Kong Med Assoc* 1994;46:118–121.

Il'nitskii VA, Manuilov NN, Meleshenkova TI: [Eye manifestations of AIDS in the population of the Republic of Burundi.] *Vestnik Oftalmol* 1990;106:58–60.

Kawe LW, Renard G, Le Hoang P, et al: [Ophthalmologic manifestations of AIDS in an African milieu: report of 45 cases.] *J Fr Ophtalmol* 1990;13:199–204.

Kestelyn P: The epidemiology of CMV retinitis in Africa. *Ocul Immunol Inflamm* 1999;7:173–177.

Kestelyn P, Van de Perre P, Rouvroy D, et al: A prospective study of the ophthalmologic findings in the acquired immune deficiency syndrome in Africa. *Am J Ophthalmol* 1985;100:230–238.

Lewallen S: Herpes zoster ophthalmicus in Malawi. *Ophthalmology* 1994;101:1801–1804.

Lewallen S: Ocular manifestations of the human immunodeficiency virus and the acquired immunodeficiency syndrome in developing countries. *Arch Ophthalmol* 1997;115:435.

Lewallen S, Courtright P: HIV and AIDS and the eye in developing countries: a review. *Arch Ophthalmol* 1997;115:1291–1295.

Lewallen S, Kumwenda J, Maher D, et al: Retinal findings in Malawian patients with AIDS. *Br J Ophthalmol* 1994;78:757–759.

Lewallen S, Shroyer KR, Keyser RB, et al: Aggressive conjunctival squamous cell carcinoma in three young Africans. *Arch Ophthalmol* 1996;114:215–218.

Lightman S: HIV/AIDS: the differing ocular manifestations in developed and developing countries. *Community Eye Health* 1995;8:17–19.

Morgan D, Jones C, Whitworth J, et al: Ocular findings in HIV-1 positive and HIV-1 negative participants in a rural population–based cohort in Uganda. *Int Ophthalmol* 1998–1999;22:183–192.

Mselle J: Fungal keratitis as an indicator of HIV infection in Africa. *Trop Doctor* 1999;29:133–135.

Muccioli C, Belfort R Jr, Lottenberg C, et al: [Ophthalmological manifestations in AIDS: evaluation of 445 patients in one year.] *Rev Assos Med Brasil* 1994;40:155–158.

Ndoye NB, Sow PS, Ba EA, et al: [Ocular manifestations of AIDS in Dakar.] *Dakar Med* 1993;38:97–100.

Tanterdtam J, Suvannagoo S, Namatra C, et al: A study of ocular manifestations in HIV patients. *Thai J Ophthalmol* 1996;10:11–20.

Umeh RE: Herpes zoster ophthalmicus and HIV infection in Nigeria. *Int J STD AIDS* 1998;9:476–479.

Van de Perre P, Bakkers E, Batungwanayo J, et al: Herpes zoster in African patients: an early manifestation of HIV infection. *Scand J Infect Dis* 1988;20:277–282.

Waddell KM, Lewallen S, Lucas SB, et al: Carcinoma of the conjunctiva and HIV infection in Uganda and Malawi. *Br J Ophthalmol* 1996;80:503–508.

From Despair to Hope

The past two decades have witnessed tremendous improvements in understanding the pathogenesis and treatment of both HIV/AIDS and its ocular complications. This is especially true in developed nations, where state-of-the-art diagnostic facilities and highly active antiretroviral therapy (HAART) are readily available. Most patients are living longer, healthier lives, with fewer blinding complications.

There are, however, still reasons to be concerned:

1. Currently, there is no cure for HIV infection. Hence, while the prevalence of AIDS and AIDS-related deaths has fallen each year since the advent of HAART in 1996, the overall prevalence of HIV has continued to rise in both North America and Europe.

2. The demographics of HIV infection are now shifting away from homosexual white men and injection drug users and toward minorities and heterosexual women, many of whom believe they are not at risk of infection, fail to use protection during sexual intercourse, and do not seek regular testing.

This increase in the prevalence of HIV infection, especially among populations that are not accustomed to being screened for HIV and so tend to present later in the course of their disease, means that, ultimately, the absolute number of complications related to HIV/AIDS will rise and

that, as eye care providers, ophthalmologists will be seeing more ocular complications of HIV disease.

The situation in the developing world is even more worrisome. The prevalence of HIV infection is increasing rapidly, particularly in Africa, India, and parts of Eastern Europe. Collectively, the number of HIV-infected patients in the developing world is well in excess of 30 million, and there appears to be no slowdown in sight. Pharmaceutical companies in North America and Europe have now agreed to make many antiretroviral agents available to HIV-infected patients in developing countries, but, in the absence of well-organized and effective treatment programs, many regions will probably provide only partial or incomplete treatment regimens. HAART, almost assuredly, will be available to very few.

The fear here, of course, is that while incomplete antiretroviral therapy may allow many patients to live longer, they may actually be at increased risk for developing HIV-related complications, because immune reconstitution cannot be effectively achieved in the absence of combination antiretroviral therapy. Patients may tend, therefore, to progress to more severe states of immunosuppression, where they will be at high risk for developing opportunistic complications, including cytomegalovirus retinitis and other blinding disorders. Some warn that this situation could even produce an epidemic blindness related to HIV/AIDS in the developing world.

Still, there are reasons to be hopeful. Governments, companies, and people at large are finally beginning to recognize the enormity of the problem, and organized responses are now being openly discussed and planned. Scientists, too, are continuing work to better understand the pathogenesis of HIV infection, to improve antiretroviral therapy, and to develop effective vaccines. Together, these efforts will undoubtedly have an enormous effect on the quality of life for millions of HIV-positive people worldwide.

SELECTED REFERENCES

Access to treatment for HIV in developing countries; statement from international seminar on access to treatment for HIV in developing countries. London, June 5–6, 1998. UK NGO AIDS Consortium Working Group on Access to Treatment for HIV in Developing Countries. *Lancet* 1998;352:1379–1380.

Beck EJ, Miners AH, Tolley K: The cost of HIV treatment and care: a global review. *Pharmacoeconomics* 2001;19:13–39.

Belfort R Jr: The ophthalmologist and the global impact of the AIDS epidemic. LV Edward Jackson Memorial Lecture. *Am J Ophthalmol* 2000; 129:1–8.

Faden R, Kass N: HIV research, ethics, and the developing world. *Am J Pub Health* 1998; 88:548–550.

Grant AD, De Cock KM: ABC of AIDS: HIV infection and AIDS in the developing world. *Br Med J* 2001;322:1475–1478.

Guex-Crosier Y, Telenti A: An epidemic of blindness: a consequence of improved HIV care? *Bull World Health Organ* 2001;79:181.

Kestelyn P: The epidemiology of CMV retinitis in Africa. *Ocul Immunol Inflamm* 1999;7:173–177.

Kestelyn PG, Cunningham ET Jr: HIV/AIDS and blindness. *Bull World Health Organ* 2001;79: 208–213.

OPHTHALMOLOGY MONOGRAPH 15
HIV/AIDS and the Eye: A Global Perspective

CME Accreditation

The American Academy of Ophthalmology is accredited by the Accreditation Council for Continuing Medical Education to provide continuing medical education for physicians.

The American Academy of Ophthalmology designates this educational activity for a maximum of 20 hours in category 1 credit toward the AMA Physician's Recognition Award. Each physician should claim only those hours of credit that he/she has actually spent in the activity.

CME Credit Report Forms

If you wish to claim CME credit for your study of this monograph, you must send this page and the following three pages (by mail or fax) to the Academy office. Please make sure to:

1. Fill in and sign the statement below.
2. Write your answers to the questions on the back of this page.
3. Complete the self-study examination and mark your answers on the answer sheet.
4. Complete the product evaluation.

Important These completed forms must be received at the Academy within 3 years of purchase.

I hereby certify that I have spent _____ (up to 20) hours of study on this monograph and that I have completed the self-study examination. (The Academy, upon request, will send you a verification of your Academy credits earned within the last 3 years.)

_____   Date _____
Signature

PLEASE PRINT

_____
Last Name   First Name   MI

_____
Mailing Address

_____
City

_____
State   ZIP Code

_____
Telephone   ID Number*

Please return the completed forms to:

American Academy of Ophthalmology
P.O. Box 7424
San Francisco, CA 94120-7424
ATTN: Clinical Education Division

*Your ID Number is located following your name on most Academy mailing labels, in your member directory, and on your monthly statement of account.

OPHTHALMOLOGY MONOGRAPH 15
HIV/AIDS and the Eye: A Global Perspective

1. Please list several ways in which your study of this monograph will affect your practice.

_____

_____

_____

_____

_____

_____

2. How can we improve this monograph to better meet your continuing medical education needs?

_____

_____

_____

_____

_____

_____

3. *Optional* Please list any topics you would like to see covered in other Academy clinical education products.

_____

_____

_____

_____

_____

_____

OPHTHALMOLOGY MONOGRAPH 15
HIV/AIDS and the Eye: A Global Perspective

Circle the letter of the response option that you regard as the "best" answer to the question.

Question	Answer					
1	a	b	c	d	e	
2	a	b	c	d	e	f
3	a	b	c	d	e	
4	a	b	c	d	e	
5	T	F				
6	a	b	c			
7	a	b	c	d		
8	a	b	c	d		
9	a	b	c	d		
10	a	b	c	d	e	
11	a	b	c	d		
12	a	b	c	d		
13	a	b	c	d	e	
14	a	b	c	d	e	
15	a	b	c	d		
16	T	F				
17	a	b	c	d	e	
18	a	b	c	d	e	
19	T	F				
20	a	b	c	d	e	
21	a	b	c	d	e	f
22	a	b	c	d		
23	T	F				
24	T	F				
25	a	b	c	d	e	f

Please complete the product evaluation on the back of this page.

107

OPHTHALMOLOGY MONOGRAPH 15
HIV/AIDS and the Eye: A Global Perspective

Please indicate your response to the statements listed below by placing the appropriate number to the left of each statement.

1 = Agree strongly

2 = Agree

3 = No opinion

4 = Disagree

5 = Disagree strongly

_____ This monograph meets its stated objectives.

_____ This monograph helped me keep current on this topic.

_____ I will apply knowledge gained from this monograph to my practice.

_____ This monograph covers topics in sufficient depth and detail.

_____ This monograph's illustrations are of sufficient number and quality.

_____ The references included in the monograph provide an appropriate amount of additional reading.

_____ The self-study examination at the end of the monograph is useful.

SELF-STUDY EXAMINATION

The self-study examination provided for each book in the Ophthalmology Monographs series is intended for use after completion of the monograph. The examination for *HIV/AIDS and the Eye: A Global Perspective* consists of 25 multiple-choice and true-false questions followed by the answers to the questions and a discussion for each answer. The Academy recommends that you not consult the answers until you have completed the entire examination.

Questions

The questions are constructed so that there is one "best" answer. Despite the attempt to avoid ambiguous selections, disagreement may occur about which selection constitutes the optimal answer. After reading a question, record your initial impression on the answer sheet.

Answers and Discussions

The "best" answer to each question is provided after the examination. The discussion that accompanies the answer is intended to help you confirm that the reasoning you used in determining the most appropriate answer was correct. If you missed a question, the discussion may help you decide whether your "error" was due to poor wording of the question or to your misinterpretation. If, instead, you missed the question because of miscalculation or failure to recall relevant information, the discussion may help fix the principle in your memory.

QUESTIONS

Chapter 1

1. Recognized risk factors for the transmission of HIV include all of the following *except*

   a. unprotected sexual intercourse

   b. injection or intravenous drug use

   c. receipt of whole blood

   d. performing an eye examination on an HIV-positive patient without the use of latex gloves

   e. breast-feeding

2. CD4$^+$ T-lymphocyte count is a reliable predictor of risk for developing various opportunistic disorders in HIV-positive patients. Match each of the following HIV-associated neoplastic and infectious disorders with the approximate CD4$^+$ T-lymphocyte count range: (**1**) <100 cells/µL; (**2**) <200 cells/µL; (**3**) <500 cells/µL.

   a. cytomegalovirus (CMV) retinitis

   b. Kaposi sarcoma

   c. tuberculosis

   d. progressive multifocal leukoencephalopathy (PML)

   e. herpes zoster ophthalmicus (HZO)

   f. toxoplasmosis

3. The Centers for Disease Control and Prevention (CDC) defines the acquired immunodeficiency syndrome (AIDS) in HIV-positive adults as any of the following *except*

   a. a CD4$^+$ T-lymphocyte count of less than 200 cells/µL

   b. cytomegalovirus (CMV) retinitis

   c. Kaposi sarcoma of the eyelid

   d. toxoplasmic retinochoroiditis

   e. cortical blindness due to progressive multifocal leukoencephalopathy (PML)

4. Current trends in the epidemiology of HIV/AIDS in North America and Europe include

   a. decreasing overall number of HIV-positive patients

   b. increasing number of HIV-positive patients among minorities and women

   c. decreasing number of patients with AIDS

   d. b and c

   e. all of the above

Chapter 2

5. The CD4 receptor on CD4⁺ T   **T**   **F**
lymphocytes is solely responsible
for virus entry and tropism for
these particular cells.

6. The term *viral latency*, as used with respect to HIV, refers to

a. the time from infection with HIV to
the development of flu-like symptoms

b. the time required for HIV to enter
CD4⁺ T lymphocytes and begin
replicating

c. the period of relatively suppressed
virus replication following infection,
but prior to the development of AIDS

7. Currently available antiretroviral agents
act by all of the following mechanisms
except

a. inhibition of the HIV enzyme protease

b. inhibition of chain elongation during
reverse transcription of HIV genomic
RNA into double-stranded proviral
DNA

c. inhibition of binding of HIV to the
CD4 receptor

d. inhibition of the HIV enzyme reverse
transcriptase

Chapter 3

8. Appropriate techniques for cleaning
tonometer tips that come in contact
with the eye include

a. a 5-minute soak in 1/10 dilution of
sodium hypochlorite (household
bleach) in 70% isopropanol

b. a 20-minute soak in fresh 3% hydrogen peroxide

c. a 50-minute soak in 70% ethanol

d. thorough wiping of the tonometer tip
with an ethanol-soaked pad

Chapter 4

9. The most common HIV-associated
malignancy is

a. squamous cell carcinoma

b. Kaposi sarcoma

c. non-Hodgkin lymphoma

d. glioblastoma

10. Initial therapy for herpes zoster ophthalmicus (HZO) in a severely immunosuppressed HIV-positive patient should
include

a. oral acyclovir 400 mg 5 times daily

b. intravenous foscarnet 90 mg/kg every
12 hours

c. oral famciclovir 500 mg 3 times daily

d. intravenous acyclovir 10 mg/kg every
8 hours

e. oral valacyclovir 1 g 3 times daily

11. All of the following statements regarding Kaposi sarcoma are true *except*

  a. It is associated with exposure to human herpes virus-8.

  b. It is relatively uncommon in Africa and Asia.

  c. It may be the presenting sign of HIV infection.

  d. It may be fatal if the lungs, gastrointestinal tract, and/or meninges are involved.

Chapter 5

12. All of the following statements about herpetic keratitis in HIV-infected patients are true *except*

  a. Both varicella zoster virus (VZV) and herpes simplex virus (HSV) may cause keratitis in HIV-positive patients.

  b. VZV keratitis occurs more commonly in HIV-positive patients as compared to immunocompetent patients.

  c. VZV keratitis occurs, but is uncommon, in HIV-positive patients with herpes zoster ophthalmicus (HZO).

  d. Skin lesions may be absent in HIV-positive patients with VZV or HSV keratitis.

13. *Candida*-associated keratitis has been reported in HIV-positive patients and appears to be associated with

  a. older age

  b. female gender

  c. prior herpetic keratitis

  d. illicit drug use

  e. oral candidiasis

14. Match the following drugs with the most appropriate adverse event reported in HIV-infected patients: (**1**) cidofovir; (**2**) rifabutin; (**3**) atovaquone; (**4**) ganciclovir; (**5**) foscarnet.

  a. hypopyon formation

  b. vortex keratopathy

  c. renal toxicity

  d. bone marrow toxicity

  e. anterior uveitis associated with ocular hypotension

Chapter 6

15. The most important reason to identify HIV retinopathy is that

  a. macular ischemia often develops and may produce profound loss of vision

  b. HIV retinopathy is a strong indicator of advanced HIV disease

  c. cytomegalovirus (CMV) retinitis often occurs at one or more of the observed cotton-wool spots

  d. prompt initiation of highly active antiretroviral therapy (HAART) may reverse formation of cotton-wool spots

16. Fulminant cytomegalovirus   **T**   **F** (CMV) retinitis is characterized by prominent retinal edema and hemorrhages and frequently advances more quickly than either the granular or the perivascular form of infection.

17. Varicella zoster virus (VZV) retinitis and herpes simplex virus (HSV) retinitis are distinguished from cytomegalovirus (CMV) retinitis by all of the following *except*

  a. rapid progression

  b. multiple foci of infection

  c. large, confluent areas of retinitis

  d. retinal vascular occlusion

  e. extensive areas of hemorrhage

18. All of the following statements about toxoplasmic retinochoroiditis in patients with HIV disease are true *except*

  a. Moderate-to-severe vitreous inflammation is often noted.

  b. Recurrences are common once specific therapy for toxoplasmosis is withdrawn.

  c. Concurrent central nervous system (CNS) involvement is observed in many patients.

  d. Many patients have a negative anti-*Toxoplasma* immunoglobin G (IgG) serum antibody titer, despite polmerase chain reaction–based evidence of active toxoplasmic retinochoroiditis.

  e. The presence of an adjacent or nearby retinochoroidal scar supports the diagnosis.

19. The rapid plasma reagin (RPR)   **T**   **F** test and the fluorescent treponemal antibody absorption (FTA-ABS) test provide equal diagnostic sensitivity with respect to ocular and central nervous system (CNS) syphilis, but the RPR test is titrated and so offers the added value of measuring disease activity.

20. All of the following statements about immune recovery uveitis (IRU) are true *except*

  a. Cystoid macular edema (CME) is the most frequent cause of vision loss related to IRU and usually results from vitreomacular traction or epiretinal membrane formation.

  b. IRU occurs only in patients who at some point have been severely immunosuppressed.

  c. Vitreous inflammation is the most common manifestation of IRU.

  d. Corticosteroids given topically, periocularly, or systemically are the primary therapy for IRU complications.

  e. While retinal neovascularization occurs as a complication of IRU, retinal ischemia or nonperfusion is usually not present.

Chapter 7

21. Homonymous visual field defects and contrast-enhancing occipital lesions in an HIV-positive patient may represent which of the following conditions?

    a. toxoplasmosis

    b. progressive multifocal leukoen-cephalopathy (PML)

    c. lymphoma

    d. tuberculosis

    e. a and b

    f. all of the above

22. Which of the following statements about cytomegalovirus (CMV) papillitis is *true*?

    a. It constitutes 1% to 2% of all CMV retinitis.

    b. Recovery of vision is improved with prolonged anti-CMV induction therapy.

    c. Vision is usually excellent at presentation because the fovea tends to be spared.

    d. An afferent pupillary defect (APD) is rarely present.

Chapter 8

23. HIV-infected children should have complete eye examinations every 3 to 4 months starting at 3 months of age.   T   F

24. Cytomegalovirus (CMV) retinitis is the most common ocular complication in HIV-infected children.   T   F

Chapter 9

25. All of the following statements about the ocular complications of HIV/AIDS in the developing world, as compared to the developed countries, are true *except*

    a. Cytomegalovirus (CMV) retinitis affects a lower percentage of patients than in North America or Europe, most probably because patients in developing countries do not live as long and so never progress to the levels of profound immunosuppression required for CMV to develop.

    b. Herpes zoster ophthalmicus (HZO), squamous cell carcinoma of the conjunctiva, and fungal keratitis all appear to occur more often in African patients with HIV disease.

    c. The prevalence of Kaposi sarcoma varies considerably from region to region and most probably reflects the prevalence of human herpes virus-8 infection.

    d. More than 90% of HIV-infected patients in the developing world are unaware of their HIV status.

    e. a, c, and d

    f. all of the above

ANSWERS AND DISCUSSIONS

Chapter 1

1. **Answer—d.** Well-recognized risk factors for the transmission of HIV include (**1**) unprotected sexual intercourse, particularly men having sex with men, sex with commercial sex workers, and sex with injection drug users; (**2**) injection drug use, especially if needle-sharing is common; (**3**) receipt of blood or blood products, solid organ or bone marrow transplantation, especially in countries where screening is poorly practiced; and (**4**) breast-feeding by an HIV-infected mother. While protective, latex gloves may be worn for any eye examination and are generally recommended if there are cuts, scratches, or dermatologic lesions on the examiner's hands or if venipuncture or invasive procedures using needles or sharp instruments are to be performed. Gloves are not generally required for performing routine eye examinations on HIV-positive patients. Hand-washing should be performed after every patient examination, however.

2. **Answer—a,d.** Necrotizing herpetic retinitis (including cytomegalovirus [CMV] retinitis, varicella zoster virus [VZV] retinitis, and herpes simplex virus [HSV] retinitis), progressive multifocal leukoencephalopathy (PML), and many other disorders, such as microsporidiosis, *Mycobacterium avium* complex infection, and retinal and conjunctival microvasculopathy, occur most commonly in the setting of severe immune depletion, once CD4$^+$ T-lymphocyte counts fall below 100 cells/µL. **c,f.** Tuberculosis and toxoplasmosis may occur at any CD4$^+$ T-lymphocyte count, but tend to occur with increased frequency at moderate levels of immune depletion, when CD4$^+$ T-lymphocyte counts are less than 200 cells/µL. **b,e.** Kaposi sarcoma and herpes zoster ophthalmicus (HZO) often occur early in the course of HIV disease, when immune depletion is mild and CD4$^+$ T-lymphocyte counts are relatively high and between 200 and 500 cells/µL. See Table 1-1.

3. **Answer—d.** While toxoplasmosis of the central nervous system (CNS) is included in the CDC 1993 revised AIDS surveillance case definition, toxoplasmic retinochoroiditis is not. A sizable proportion of HIV-positive patients with ocular toxoplasmosis either have or will develop CNS toxoplasmosis, however. Additional conditions included in the CDC 1993 revised AIDS surveillance case definition are listed in Table 1-2. Children tend to have higher CD4$^+$ T-lymphocyte counts than do adults; for this reason, a cutoff of 750 cells/µL is used for children under 1 year of age, and a cutoff of 500 cells/µL is used for children 1 to 5 years of age. The adult definition of 200 cells/µL is used for children 6 years of age and older.

4. **Answer—d.** The number of HIV-positive patients in North America and Europe continues to increase each year, particularly among minorities and women. The introduction of highly active antiretroviral therapy (HAART) in 1996 has allowed many patients in developed countries to live longer without progression to AIDS.

Chapter 2

5. **Answer—F.** Although the HIV envelope glycoprotein gp120^{env} binds to the CD4 receptor with high affinity, cellular entry requires the presence of a coreceptor, such as the chemokine receptor CCR5 or CXCR4. Patients who lack such coreceptors are resistant to infection with HIV.

6. **Answer—c.** It should be noted, however, that even during periods of viral latency, patients typically have 10^3 to 10^6 copies of HIV RNA per milliliter of plasma, even in the absence of highly active antiretroviral therapy (HAART). This period of viral latency corresponds to the period of clinical latency shown in Figure 1-2, which may last 10 years or more in untreated patients.

7. **Answer—c.** HIV protease inhibitors bind to, and inhibit, HIV protease, which cleaves *gag-pol* precursors into the mature structural proteins that are required for virus assembly. Nucleoside analogs competitively inhibit DNA chain elongation. Nonnucleoside reverse-transcriptase inhibitors (NNRTI) bind to, and inhibit, HIV reverse transcriptase. All three classes of agents are used clinically. Combined use of three or more such agents is referred to as *highly active antiretroviral therapy* (HAART). Inhibitors of HIV binding to the CD4 receptor are currently being developed, but have not yet been approved for use in humans. See Section 2-8, "Antiretroviral Agents," for specific agents.

Chapter 3

8. **Answer—a,b.** Appropriate techniques include (**1**) a 5- to 50-minute soak in bleach in either 70% isopropanol or 70% ethanol; or (**2**) a 5- to 50-minute soak in 3% hydrogen peroxide. These solutions need to made fresh daily because concentrations change quickly with evaporation. Isopropanol or ethanol alone, either in solution or on an impregnated pad, is inadequate.

Chapter 4

9. Answer—b. Kaposi sarcoma is the most common HIV-associated malignancy, although it occurs much less frequently in Africa and Asia as compared to North America, Europe, and portions of South America. Squamous cell carcinoma and non-Hodgkin lymphoma occur with increased frequency in HIV-infected patients, but are still relatively uncommon. Glioblastoma appears not to occur with increased frequency in HIV-positive patients.

10. Answer—d. Intravenous acyclovir is the standard therapy for herpes zoster ophthalmicus (HZO) in severely immunosuppressed HIV-positive patients, is typically given for 1 week, and is then followed by maintenance therapy with either oral acyclovir (800 mg 5 times daily) or oral famciclovir (500 mg 3 times daily). Both oral acyclovir and oral famciclovir may be used to treat HZO in immunocompetent patients. Intravenous foscarnet or ganciclovir may be used alone or in combination with intravenous acyclovir in patients who fail to respond to initial therapy. Valacyclovir should be avoided in severely immunosuppressed patients because of isolated reports of thrombocytopenic purpuric/hemolytic uremic syndrome. The efficacy of oral valganciclovir in the treatment of HZO is unknown, although drug levels appear to be comparable to, or better than, those achieved with intravenous ganciclovir.

11. Answer—d. While Kaposi sarcoma of the lung, gastrointestinal tract, and other visceral organs does occur and may be fatal if left untreated, meningeal involvement has not been reported. The reason for the lower prevalence of Kaposi sarcoma in Africa and Asia is unknown, although lower rates of human herpes virus-8 infection in these regions may account, at least in part, for observed differences.

Chapter 5

12. Answer—c. Varicella zoster virus (VZV) keratitis occurs in approximately one third of HIV-positive patients with herpes zoster ophthalmicus (HZO).

13. Answer—d. Illicit drug use has been noted as a frequent behavior in HIV-infected patients with *Candida*-associated keratitis.

14. Answer—e. Cidofovir produces anterior uveitis in up to 50% of patients and may be associated with ocular hypotension. **a.** Rifabutin, which is used to treat *Mycobacterium avium* complex infections, produces severe iritis, which may result in hypopyon formation, in up to one third of patients. **b.** Atovaquone has been associated with vortex keratopathy in isolated patients. **d.** Ganciclovir may cause neutropenia. **c.** Foscarnet has been associated with nephropathy.

Chapter 6

15. **Answer—b.** HIV retinopathy occurs only in HIV-infected patients with low CD4$^+$ T-lymphocyte counts and is therefore an important indicator of advanced disease. While macular ischemia has been observed in HIV-positive patients and may be pathophysiologically related to HIV retinopathy, loss of vision related to enlargement of the foveal avascular zone appears to be uncommon. Cytomegalovirus (CMV) retinitis can occur either together with or following the development of HIV retinopathy, but its location appears to be largely unrelated to the location of cotton-wool spots, which resolve over time with or without the initiation of highly active antiretroviral therapy (HAART).

16. **Answer—F.** While retinal edema and hemorrhages characterize fulminant cytomegalovirus (CMV) retinitis, rates of progression and recurrence appear to be similar for all forms of infection.

17. **Answer—e.** Hemorrhages may be seen in association with any necrotizing herpetic retinitis, including cytomegalovirus (CMV) retinitis. While polymerase chain reaction–based analysis of ocular specimens is the best way to distinguish varicella zoster virus (VZV) retinitis from herpes simplex virus (HSV) retinitis, prior or concurrent herpes zoster ophthalmicus (HZO) or VZV dermatitis may sometimes be elicited in patients with VZV retinitis, whereas a history of encephalitis may be noted before or together with the onset of HSV retinitis.

18. **Answer—d.** While a false-negative anti-*Toxoplasma* immunoglobin G (IgG) serum antibody titer may occur in HIV-positive patients with active toxoplasmic retinochoroiditis, it is uncommon.

19. **Answer—F.** While both the rapid plasma reagin (RPR) test and the Venereal Disease Research Laboratory (VDRL) test are titrated and provide an indirect measure of disease activity, both the RPR and the VDRL are negative in up to 30% of patients with ocular or central nervous system (CNS) syphilis. The fluorescent treponemal antibody absorption (FTA-ABS) test and the microhemagglutination assay for *Treponema pallidum* (MHA-TP), in contrast, have greater than 90% sensitivity.

20. **Answer—a.** While cystoid macular edema (CME) is the most common cause of vision loss in HIV-positive patients with immune recovery uveitis (IRU) and may result from, or be exacerbated by, vitreomacular traction or epiretinal membrane formation, IRU-related CME occurs most frequently in the absence of such vitreoretinal interface changes. Corticosteroids are the primary therapy for IRU-related complications, but their effectiveness is limited in many patients. Reversal of vision loss due to vitreomacular traction or epiretinal membrane formation requires vitreoretinal surgery.

Chapter 7

21. **Answer—f.** While toxoplasmosis is the most common cause for a contrast-enhancing occipital lesion in HIV-positive patients, each of the disorders listed may produce such changes. Cerebrospinal fluid (CSF) analysis and biopsy are usually indicated.

22. **Answer—b.** From 3 to 6 weeks of anti-CMV induction therapy is recommended because this regimen may improve recovery of vision. CMV papillitis constitutes 5% to 10% of all CMV retinitis and is almost always associated with an afferent pupillary defect (APD) and moderate-to-severe loss of vision. An associated serous retinal detachment may be present and often flattens with anti-CMV therapy.

Chapter 8

23. **Answer—F.** Unless otherwise indicated, annual eye examinations suffice. More frequent examinations, perhaps every 3 to 4 months, should be performed if (**1**) visual signs or symptoms develop; (**2**) cytomegalovirus (CMV) is cultured from the blood, urine, or nasopharynx; (**3**) nonocular CMV infection develops; (**4**) an AIDS-defining illness occurs; or (**5**) the total CD4+ cell count falls below immune category 3 for age, severe suppression (see Table 8-1).

24. **Answer—T.** Although cytomegalovirus (CMV) retinitis is less common in HIV-positive children than in HIV-positive adults (affecting 2% to 4% of HIV-positive children), it is still the most frequent complication. Treatment strategies are similar for children and adults.

Chapter 9

25. **Answer—f.** All of the statements about the ocular complications of HIV/AIDS in the developing world are true.

INDEX

NOTE: An *f* following a page number indicates a figure, and a *t* following a page number indicates a table. Drugs are listed under their generic names; when a drug trade name is listed, the reader is referred to the generic name.

A

Abacavir, 25
ABC. *See* Abacavir
Acquired immunodeficiency syndrome (AIDS),
    1, 5*f*, 6. *See also* HIV infection/AIDS
    definitions of, 9, 9*t*
    in children, 9, 87
Acute angle-closure glaucoma, 50–51
Acute retinal necrosis (ARN), 62
Acyclovir
    corneal toxicity of, 49
    for herpes simplex virus (HSV) infection
        keratitis, 47
        retinitis, 64
    for varicella zoster virus (VZV) infection
        (herpes zoster ophthalmicus [HZO])
        adnexal, 36
        keratitis, 46
        retinitis, 63
Adnexal manifestations of HIV infection, 35–41.
    See also specific type
    conjunctival microvasculopathy, 40, 40*f*
    conjunctivitis, 40, 40*f*
    cutaneous lymphoma, 38
    herpes zoster ophthalmicus (HZO), 35–36, 35*f*
    hypertrichosis (trichomegaly), 39–40, 39*f*
    Kaposi sarcoma, 36–38, 37*f*
    molluscum contagiosum, 38, 39*f*
    preseptal cellulitis, 41
    squamous cell carcinoma, 38, 39*f*
    trichomegaly (hypertrichosis), 39–40, 39*f*
Africa
    HIV infection/AIDS epidemiology in
        in North Africa, 10*f*, 12*t*
        in sub-Saharan Africa, 10*f*, 11*f*, 12*t*, 15–16
    HIV infection/AIDS manifestations in, 97–99,
        98*f*, 99*f*

Agenerase. *See* Amprenavir
AIDS. *See* Acquired immunodeficiency syndrome
AIDS dementia, 76–77
Albendazole, for microsporidial keratitis, 48
Amphotericin B, for cryptococcal meningitis, 78
Amprenavir, 26
Anal intercourse, sexual transmission of HIV
    and, 2
Angle-closure glaucoma, 50–51
Anterior segment, HIV manifestations in, 45–53.
        See also specific type
    angle-closure glaucoma, 50–51
    anterior uveitis, 49–50, 50*f*
    corneal drug toxicity, 49
    infectious keratitis, 46–48, 47*f*, 48*f*
    keratoconjunctivitis sicca, 45–46, 45*f*
Anterior uveitis, 49–50, 50*f*
    in varicella zoster virus (VZV) infection
        (herpes zoster ophthalmicus [HZO]),
        46, 49
Antibody tests for HIV, 8
    for blood/blood products, transmission
        prevention and, 3
    in newborns, 87
Antiretroviral therapy, 25–26. *See also specific*
        agent and Highly active antiretroviral
        therapy
    current status of, 103–104
    mother-to-infant transmission affected by, 3
    postexposure, 4

ARN (acute retinal necrosis), 62
Asia
    HIV infection/AIDS epidemiology in
        in Central Asia, 10*f*, 12*t*, 14
        in East Asia, 10*f*, 11*f*, 12*t*
        in South/Southeast Asia, 10*f*, 11*f*, 12*t*, 15
    HIV infection/AIDS manifestations in, 99–100
Aspergillus
    orbital cellulitis caused by, 41
    retinitis caused by, 66
Atovaquone
    for cerebral toxoplasmosis, 78
    corneal toxicity of, 49
    for toxoplasmic retinochoroiditis, 65
Australia, HIV infection/AIDS epidemiology in,
        10*f*, 11*f*, 12*t*
Azathioprine, for toxoplasmic retinochoroiditis,
        65
AZT. *See* Zidovudine

B
Bacterial keratitis, 48
Bacterial retinitis, 65–66, 65*f*
Barrier precautions, HIV transmission preven-
        tion and, 29
Bartonella henselae, neuroretinitis caused by, 66
Bisexual men, sexual transmission of HIV and, 2
Blindness, cortical, 83
Blood/blood products, in HIV transmission, 3
Brazil, HIV infection/AIDS epidemiology in, 15
Breast-feeding, HIV transmission and, 3
Brolene. *See* Propamidine
Budding, in HIV virion assembly, 25

C
CA (capsid protein), 20, 22, 22*f*
Candida, retinitis caused by, 66
Capsaicin, for postherpetic neuralgia, 46
Capsid protein (CA), 20, 22, 22*f*
Cardiopulmonary resuscitation, HIV transmis-
        sion prevention and, 30
Caribbean, HIV infection/AIDS epidemiology
        in, 10*f*, 11*f*, 12*t*, 15
CCR5 HIV coreceptor, 23
CD4+ T-lymphocyte count. *See also* CD4+ T
        lymphocytes
    in AIDS definition, 9
        in children, 87
    cerebral toxoplasmosis and, 77
    conjunctival microvasculopathy and, 40
    cytomegalovirus (CMV) papillitis and, 82
    cytomegalovirus (CMV) retinitis and, 56
    dementia and, 76
    herpes zoster ophthalmicus (HZO) and, 36
    highly active antiretroviral therapy (HAART)
        affecting, 6–7, 6*f*
    in latent phase of HIV infection, 5*f*, 6
    mother-to-infant transmission and, 3
    opportunistic disorders and, 7, 7*t*, 9
        in children, 88, 88*t*
    primary central nervous system lymphoma
        and, 80
    in primary infection, 5, 5*f*
    progressive multifocal leukoencephalopathy
        (PML) and, 79
CD4+ T lymphocytes. *See also* CD4+ T-lympho-
        cyte count
    HIV infection of, 1, 2*f*
        molecular mechanisms of, 19, 23, 24*f*
        viral latency and, 24
CDC. *See* Centers for Disease Control and
        Prevention
Cellular attachment, HIV, 23
Cellular entry, HIV, 23
Cellulitis, orbital, 41, 41*f*, 42

K

Kaletra. *See* Lipinovir with ritonavir
Kaposi sarcoma
  adnexal, 36–38, 37*f*
  orbital, 41
Keratitis, infectious, 46–48, 47*f*, 48*f*. *See also*
      specific type
  bacterial, 48
  cytomegalovirus (CMV) causing, 47–48
  fungal, 48
  herpes simplex virus (HSV) causing, 46–47,
      47*f*
  microsporidial, 48, 49*f*
  varicella zoster virus (VZV) causing, 46, 47*f*
Keratoconjunctivitis sicca, 45–46, 45*f*
Keratopathy
drug toxicity causing, 49
epithelial, microsporidial, 49*f*

L

Lamivudine, 25
Latency
  clinical, 5–6, 5*f*
    neurologic symptoms during, 75–76
  viral, 24
Latex condoms, HIV transmission prevention
      and, 2
Latin America
  HIV infection/AIDS epidemiology in, 10*f*, 11*f*,
      12*t*, 15
  HIV infection/AIDS manifestations in, 100,
      100*f*
Lentivirus, HIV as, 20
Leukoencephalopathy, progressive multifocal
      (PML), 79, 79*f*
  visual field defects and cortical vision loss and,
      83
Lipid bilayer, of HIV virion, 22–23, 22*f*
Lipinovir with ritonavir, 26

Lymphoma
  adnexal, 38
  central nervous system, primary, 80, 81*f*
  intraocular, 66
  oculomotor nerve paresis and, 84
  orbital, 41, 41*f*, 42
  papillitis caused by, 82, 83*f*

M

MA (matrix protein), 20, 22, 22*f*
  in DNA integration, 23
Macrophages, HIV infection of, 75
Mask, HIV transmission prevention and, 29
Matrix protein (MA), 20, 22, 22*f*
  in DNA integration, 23
Memory T cells, viral latency and, 24
Meningitis
  cryptococcal, 78–79, 78*f*
    in Asia, 99–100
      oculomotor nerve paresis and, 83
  oculomotor nerve paresis and, 83
  as primary HIV disorder, 76
  syphilitic, 79–80
Methicillin, for staphylococcal preseptal cellu-
      litis, 41
Mexico, HIV infection/AIDS epidemiology in,
      15
MHA-TP (microhemagglutination assay for
      Treponema pallidum)
  for neurosyphilis, 80
  for ocular syphilis, 66
Microglial cells, HIV infection of, 75